OPERATIVE MANAGEMENT OF LOWER EXTREMITY FRACTURES IN CHILDREN

Edited by Robert N. Hensinger, MD
Professor of Surgery
Section of Orthopaedics
University of Michigan
Ann Arbor, Michigan

Contributors
James H. Beaty, MD
Dennis P. Devito, MD
Robert N. Hensinger, MD
James R. Kasser, MD
Randall T. Loder, MD
George T. Rab, MD

Series Editor
Herbert Kaufer, MD

American Academy of Orthopaedic Surgeons
222 South Prospect Avenue
Park Ridge, Illinois 60068

American Academy of Orthopaedic Surgeons

OPERATIVE MANAGEMENT OF LOWER EXTREMITY FRACTURES IN CHILDREN

Executive Director:
Thomas C. Nelson

Director of Communications and Publications:
Mark W. Wieting

Assistant Director, Publications:
Marilyn L. Fox, PhD

Senior Editor:
Bruce Davis

Production Manager:
Loraine Edwalds

Production Editor:
Monica M. Trocker

Publications Secretary:
Geraldine Dubberke

The American Academy of Orthopaedic Surgeons Monograph Series is dedicated to Wendy O. Schmidt, American Academy of Orthopaedic Surgeons senior medical editor, 1987–1991.

Library of Congress Cataloging-in-Publication Data

Operative Management of Lower Extremity Fractures in Children/edited by Robert N. Hensinger, MD

ISBN: 0–89203–058–5

CONTRIBUTORS

James H. Beaty, MD
Associate Professor of Orthopaedic Surgery
The Campbell Clinic–University of Tennessee
Memphis, Tennessee

Dennis P. Devito, MD
Pediatric Orthopaedic Surgeon
Scottish Rite Children's Medical Center
Atlanta, Georgia

Robert N. Hensinger, MD
Professor of Surgery
Section of Orthopaedics
University of Michigan
Ann Arbor, Michigan

James R. Kasser, MD
Associate Chief of Orthopaedic Surgery
Children's Hospital
Boston, Massachusetts

Randall T. Loder, MD
Assistant Professor of Surgery
Section of Orthopaedics
University of Michigan
Ann Arbor, Michigan

George T. Rab, MD
Professor of Orthopaedic Surgery
University of California–Davis
Sacramento, California

PREFACE

There has been considerable change in the management of children's fractures over the past 20 years. Previous texts have encouraged nonoperative management and avoidance of surgical intervention except in the most extreme circumstances. In 1955, Walter Blount, in his book *Fractures in Children*, stressed the need for closed management because of the many problems and complications experienced from operative treatment. With the development of pediatric orthopaedics as a specialty, our experiences have broadened and we have gained considerable insight into the pathophysiology and anatomy of children. We have a greater appreciation of the limits of fracture remodeling, and the devastating problems that occur from premature growth arrests. Similarly, more children are surviving severe and violent injuries, which has forced us to reconsider many of our previous management recommendations. Immediate reduction and stabilization of certain injuries, particularly those that involve the physis, epiphysis, and joint surfaces, has resulted in improved results in bone growth and joint mechanics. Similarly, the polytraumatized child, the child with head injuries, and those with serious neurovascular and soft-tissue injuries from burns, lawnmower accidents, and propeller injuries have had their care significantly improved and the incidence of complications reduced by timely operative intervention.

Authors of this monograph are James H. Beaty, MD, hip and acetabulum; George T. Rab, MD, femur; James R. Kasser, MD, knee; Dennis P. Devito, MD, tibia; and Randall T. Loder, MD, foot and ankle. These authors wish to emphasize that there are still many fractures and injuries of the lower extremities that can be adequately treated by conservative techniques. Our intent in this monograph is to identify those circumstances in which the results can be improved by operative intervention. Also, the range of techniques involved is reviewed and illustrated and the pitfalls and complications are discussed in detail.

ROBERT N. HENSINGER, MD

INTRODUCTION

Polytrauma is the primary cause of serious lower extremity injuries in childhood, with automobiles accounting for 45% (passenger, 15%; pedestrian, 30%) and falls 40%.[1] Importantly, over 100,000 children are permanently crippled and 15,000 die (one half of the deaths in those younger than 15 years of age) from polytrauma each year.[2] Of polytraumatized children, 50% have an associated head injury, and 30% to 50% have an extremity injury. These statistics substantiate Waddell's finding of a triad of injuries, which includes: (1) A fracture of the femur, (2) an injury to the thorax or upper extremity on the same side, and (3) a contralateral head injury. Concomitant injuries to the spine (42%), chest (25%), and abdomen (15%) are associated with the highest incidence of mortality.[1] Only a small percentage of all head injuries result in death; however, they occur with greater frequency, and, thus, they account for the highest number of deaths in childhood trauma. Extremity fractures alone account for only 4% of the mortality, but they are the most frequent cause of severe injuries in children.[1,2]

Children with polytrauma have a survival rate higher than that of similarly injured adults. Residual morbidity in the surviving child is usually related to orthopaedic and neurologic injuries.[3] Thus, the initial management of the injured child must also be concerned with obtaining a satisfactory long-term result with a minimum of complications. Limited management of childhood trauma, such as accepting less than optimal alignment of a fracture because of its severity or because of associated injuries, will frequently be regretted.[3-5] Similarly, follow-up until maturity, especially if a leg-length discrepancy is anticipated, is recommended for all lower extremity fractures in children.

INITIAL EVALUATION

As with the adult, the injured child should be evaluated as to the status of the airway, the presence of hemorrhage and shock, and the state of consciousness. Because vomiting is common in children, a nasogastric tube or equipment for suction should be available. It is essential to conduct a careful search for internal injuries and to assess the severity of associated soft-tissue injuries. Cervical spine injuries are frequently associated with injury to the head and face. Children who are unconscious or who have neurologic findings and/ or neck pain require immediate cervical protection until appropriate radiographs can be obtained to rule out a cervical injury.

General supportive measures are the same as with an adult and should start at once with routine resuscitation: (1) Maintenance of the airway, which may require intubation; (2) insertion of an intravenous line of sufficient caliber to allow rapid transfusion (intra-osseous infusion can be used if intravenous access is limited);[6] (3) maintenance of arterial blood pressure, achieved with early infusion of Ringer's solution followed by properly matched blood; (4) insertion of a nasogastric tube; (5) cardiac monitoring; and (6) intracranial pressure monitoring for patients suspected of increased intracranial pressure.[7]

The child's blood volume, which relates directly to body weight, is approximately 40 ml per pound, regardless of age or size. Pulse rates gradually decrease with age; the upper limits of normal are 160 per minute in infants, 140 in preschool children, and 120 in older children. The normal systolic blood pressure is 80 mm of mercury plus twice the age (in years), and the normal diastolic pressure is two-thirds of the systolic pressure. Normal urine output averages 1 ml per pound per hour in small children and 0.5 ml in older children.

After medical stabilization has been achieved, extremity fractures should be splinted and dislocations reduced to minimize further soft-tissue injury and pain. If a child is in shock from hemorrhage, the chest, abdomen, and pelvis should be first suspected as the source. Shock is rarely caused by fracture alone, unless there are multiple fractures. An isolated femur fracture accounts for about 15% to 20% loss in blood volume, and only a third of such patients have a slight fall in hematocrit.[8,9] Abdominal injuries are often associated with fractures of the pelvis, fractures of the

1

TABLE 1
Pediatric Trauma Scale

	Category (Score)		
Component	**+2**	**+1**	**−1**
Size	>20 kg	10–20 kg	<10 kg
Airway	Normal	Maintainable	Unmaintainable
Systolic blood pressure	>90 mm Hg	50–90 mm Hg	<50 mm Hg
Central Nervous System	Awake	Obtunded/LOC	Coma/decerebrate
Skeletal	None	Closed fracture	Open/multiple fracture
Cutaneous	None	Minor	Major/penetrating

*If no proper size blood pressure cuff is available, assign +2 for pulse palpable at wrist, +1 for pulse palpable at groin, −1 for no pulse.

TABLE 2
Glasgow Coma Scale

Scale	Eye Opening	Best Motor Response	Best Verbal Response
6		Obeys commands	
5		Localizes pain	Oriented
4	Spontaneous	Withdraws	Confused
3	To speech	Flexes to pain	Inappropriate
2	To pain	Extends to pain	2-Incomprehensible
1	None	None	None

(Reproduced with permission from Hahn YS, Shyung C, Barthel MJ, et al: Head injuries in children under 36 months of age. *Child Nerv Syst* 1988;4:34–40.)

transverse processes of the vertebrae, or seatbelt injuries to the lumbar spine.

The Pediatric Trauma Scale (Table 1) is used at the scene for a quick and easy evaluation of injury severity and mortality potential or is used in the emergency room as a triage tool.[10] The revised trauma score for all ages is also acceptable.[11] The Glasgow Coma Scale (Table 2) has been difficult to use to assess the head-injured child under 5 years of age. Thus, it has been modified to recognize the expected normal verbal and motor responses of the very young child (Table 3).[7,12] The Modified Injury Severity Scale (Table 4), an excellent tool for retrospective studies, includes the face and neck, chest, abdomen, and the musculoskeletal and neurologic organ systems. The assessment of risk factors using the modified injury severity scale for children with multiple trauma can be useful in predicting morbidity

TABLE 3
Pediatric modification

Best Verbal Response	Adelaide Scale	Children's Memorial Scale	
5	Oriented	Smiles, oriented to sound, follows objects, interacts	
		Crying	**Interaction**
4	Words (>12 months)	Consolable	Inappropriate
3	Vocal sounds (6–12 months)	Inconsistently consolable	Moaning
2	Cries	Inconsolable	Irritable, restless
1	None	No response	No response

(Reproduced with permission from Reilly PL, Simpson DA, Sprod R, et al: Assessing the conscious level in infants and young children: A paediatric version of the Glasgow Coma Scale. *Child Nerv Syst* 1988;4:30–33.)

and mortality and aids in selecting the most appropriate method for management.[3,13,14]

Radiologic Evaluation of the Cervical Spine

Virtually every polytrauma patient arrives at the hospital on a backboard with the cervical spine immobilized. Even if the patient is alert, cooperative, and does not complain of neck pain, ambulance protocols dictate spinal immobilization. Thus, the emergency-room physician must determine whether or not radiographic evaluation of the cervical spine is necessary. Guidelines have been established for evaluating adults. Cervical spine radiographs are routinely required for patients who complain of neck pain, are intoxicated, or have decreased mentation. For initial screening, lateral, anteroposterior, odontoid, and oblique radiographs are recommended. If the patient is medically unstable, a simple cross-table lateral radiograph will suffice until the patient's condition permits a complete evaluation. Because the false negative rate for a single cross-table lateral radiograph is 23% to 36%, it is essential to follow-up with a complete cervical study.[15,16]

Rachesky and associates,[17] after reviewing a large series of injured children, concluded that cervical spine radiographs were indicated if the child complained of neck pain or if there was head or facial trauma associated with a motor vehicle accident (Fig. 1, *left*). Whenever the diagnosis of a cervical spine injury is made, a careful examination should be made of the remaining cervical spine, because in children there is a high incidence (24%) of multiple level injury.[18] Further imaging, particularly flexion-extension lateral radiographs, may be required to assess spinal stability. Computed tomography should not be used as a screening tool, but, rather, to further characterize suspicious areas found on plain films.[19] Computed tomography is recommended for all C1 fractures and in planning treatment of cervical spinal injuries.[19]

Although adults may be positioned safely supine on a flat backboard to immobilize the cervical spine, small children are different. Because young children have disproportionately larger heads, they are at risk of developing kyphosis and anterior translation of the upper cervical segment in an unstable fracture pattern (Fig. 1, *right*). I recommend positioning children younger than 6 years of age with a split mattress technique to elevate the thorax 2 to 4 cm and to lower the occiput.[20] Note that this immobilization protocol tends to reduce displaced fractures and make their recognition more difficult.

Classification of Epiphyseal Fractures

The Salter-Harris classification (Fig. 2) is probably the most widely used classification

TABLE 4
Modified Injury Severity Scale (MISS)

Body area	Score on Scale				
	1 **Minor**	**2** **Moderate**	**3** **Severe, not life-threatening**	**4** **Severe, life-threatening**	**5** **Critical, survival uncertain**
Face and neck	Abrasion or contusions of ocular apparatus or lid; vitreous or conjunctival hemorrhage; fractured teeth	Undisplaced facial bone fracture; laceration of eye or disfiguring laceration; retinal detachment	Loss of eye, avulsion of optic nerve; displaced bone fracture; blowout fracture of orbit; cervical spine fracture	Bone or soft tissue injury with minor airway obstruction; cervical spine fracture with quadriplegia	Injuries with major airway obstruction
Chest	Muscle ache or chest wall stiffness	Simple rib or sternal fracture	Multiple rib fractures; hemothorax or pneumothorax; diaphragmatic rupture; pulmonary contusion	Open chest wounds; pneumo-mediastinum; myocardial contusion	Tracheal lacerations; hemomediastinum; aortic laceration; myocardial laceration or rupture
Abdomen	Muscle ache; seat belt abrasion	Major abdominal wall contusion	Contusion of abdominal organs; retroperitoneal hematoma; extraperitoneal bladder rupture; thoracic or lumbar spine fracture	Minor laceration of abdominal organs; intraperitoneal bladder rupture; thoracic or lumbar spine fracture with paraplegia	Rupture or severe laceration of abdominal vessels or organs
Musculo-skeletal	Minor sprains; simple fractures and dislocations	Open fractures of digits; non-displaced long bone or pelvic fractures	Displaced long bone or multiple hand or foot fractures; single open long bone fracture; pelvic fractures with displacement; laceration of major nerves or vessels	Multiple closed long bone fractures; traumatic amputation	Multiple open long bone fractures
Neural*	GCS 15	GCS 13–14	GCS 9–12	GCS 5–8 or GCS 9–12 with mass lesion; impaired or absent pupillary response; impaired or absent oculocephalic or oculovestibular response	GCS <4 or GCS 5–8 with mass lesion; impaired or absent pupillary response; impaired or absent oculocephalic or oculovestibular response

*GCS = Glasgow Coma Scale.
(Reproduced with permission from Loder RT: Pediatric polytrauma: Orthopaedic care and hospital course. *J Orthop Trauma* 1987;1:48–54.)

FIGURE 1
Left, Supine lateral radiograph of a 6-year-old child with severe skull and cervical fracture who was struck by an automobile. **Right**, Note the unstable tear-drop fracture of the body of C1 with kyphosis at the fracture site (*arrow*). Adults may be safely positioned supine on a flat backboard to immobilize the cervical spine, but small children are different. Many children have disproportionately large heads and in an unstable fracture pattern are at risk of developing kyphosis and anterior translation of the upper cervical segment. Children younger than 6 years of age should be positioned using a split mattress technique to elevate the thorax 2–4 cm and lower the occiput. (Reproduced with permission from Herzenberg JE, Hensinger RN: Pediatric cervical spine injuries. *Traum Q* 1989;5:73–81.)

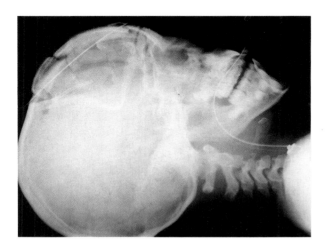
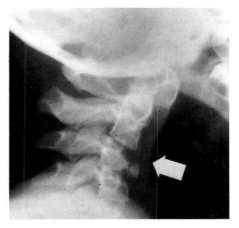

scheme and is based primarily on the radiographic appearance of the fracture. In the Salter-Harris type I injury, the epiphysis completely separates from the metaphysis without evidence of a metaphyseal fragment. This injury tends to occur in younger children, and the periosteum is usually attached over a large portion of the metaphysis. In most cases, the displacement can be reduced closed and the injury heals quickly with good results.[21]

The type II injury is the most common fracture pattern. The fracture travels through the physis transversely and then exits through the metaphysis, leaving a triangular portion of the metaphysis attached to the epiphyseal plate ("Thurston-Holland" fragment). In epiphyses, such as the distal radius, with small cross-sectional areas, satisfactory healing can be expected following closed reduction. In those of large area, however, such as the distal femur, significant growth plate disturbance is common, leading to leg length discrepancy (56%) and angulation (26%).[22]

The type III injury is an intra-articular fracture of the epiphysis and is the reverse of the type II. The fracture traverses the epiphyseal plate and then propagates or extends through the epiphysis. The medial malleolus and distal femur are the most common locations. This type of fracture requires exact anatomic reduction to restore the integrity of the joint and to avoid growth-plate arrest.

In the type IV injury, the metaphysis and epiphysis, including the articular surface, are split. The fracture travels longitudinally through the bone, crosses the physis, and exits through the metaphysis.[22,23] Nearly all type IV injuries require surgical reduction, because there is a strong propensity for early migration or displacement with resultant asymmetric healing of the fracture fragments and increased potential for late deformity.

The type V is a crushing injury to the epiphysis with very little displacement; it may not be apparent on the initial films. This crushing eventually leads to early bony bridging with

FIGURE 2

Salter-Harris Classification. This classification, based primarily on the radiographic appearance of the fracture, is the most widely used. Type I, epiphysis completely separates from the metaphysis without evidence of metaphyseal fragment. Type II, the fracture traverses the physis transversely and then exits through the metaphysis, leaving the triangular portion of the metaphysis attached to the epiphyseal plate (Thurston-Holland fragment). Type III, an interarticular fracture of the epiphysis, is the reverse of type II. The fracture traverses the epiphyseal plate and propagates or extends through the epiphysis. In type IV, the metaphysis and epiphysis, including the articular surface, are split. The fracture travels longitudinally through the bone, crosses the physis, and exits through the metaphysis. Type V is a crushing injury to the epiphysis with very little displacement. This may not be apparent on initial films. Type VI (Rang) is a localized injury to the perichondral ring. The reparative process may lead to osseous bridge and rapid development of an angular deformity. (Reproduced with permission from Rang ML: *The Growth Plate and Its Disorders.* Edinburgh, E & S Livingstone Ltd., 1969, p 139.)

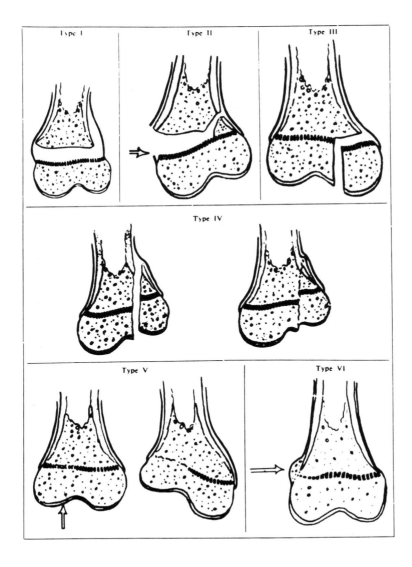

secondary angular deformity or growth arrest. Rang[24] has suggested adding a type VI injury, injury to the perichondral ring. This pattern is secondary to local injury and/or the reparative process leading to an osseous bridge and the rapid development of an angular deformity.

Ogden[25] has expanded the simpler Salter-Harris classification into a more complex system by adding epiphyseal injuries that do not involve the metaphysis and by including more extensive classification patterns (particularly intra-articular injuries) that reflect the wide variation of children's injuries (Fig. 3).

Classification of Open Fractures

For open fractures, the same classification system used for adults generally applies for children (Table 5), although the wound size must be decreased proportionally. In children, the incidence of vascular injury (5%) and compartment syndrome (5%) is similar to that reported in adults.[26] In children with grade II or III injuries, the fractures should be managed using the same guidelines for severe soft-tissue injuries as are used for adults. Thoroughly debride all necrotic and traumatized tissue with copious irrigation and leave the wounds open. Plan to redebride in the operating room every two days until clean wounds are achieved. Broad spectrum cephalosporins are routinely given to all children, and the addition of penicillin is recommended for farm-related injuries.[26]

ASSOCIATED INJURIES

Head Injury

Ninety percent of children with head injuries recover from coma in less than 48 hours. Of children who were in deep coma (score 5 to 7 on the Glasgow scale), 84% eventually are able to walk freely, and initially one must assume a full neurological recovery.[27] Both Ziv and Rang[5] and Loder[13] emphasize the importance of using the Glasgow Coma Scale (Table 3) for selecting those fractures that should be fixed. Patients with a Glasgow Score over 5 (neural Modified Injury Severity Scale score of 4 or less) tend to recover fully. If the patient has not recovered in three days, the fracture should be fixed (in children older than 5 years of age) as if recovery will be complete.[5,13,27] We recommend rigid fixation of all long bone fractures to aid in nursing care and rehabilitation efforts. Muscle spasticity in the first few days can often displace or angulate fractures immobilized in casts and can lead to overriding of those in traction.[27,28] Conservative management of fractures in these children results in healing but has an unacceptable incidence of malunion, angulation, and shortening.[27] Skin insensitivity combined with disorientation may result in skin breakdown with the potential for secondary osteomyelitis.[27]

If the child is to be moved for such special studies as computed tomography and magnetic resonance imaging (MRI), requires extensive dressing changes or multiple debridements in the operating room, or must go to the whirlpool for burns treatment, the fractures should be stabilized, because manipulation of the fracture can increase the intracranial pressure. In children with acute quadriplegia or paraplegia, fracture fixation decreases the incidence of skin problems and pressure sores from cast immobilization and avoids the need for external support, which can compromise nursing and rehabilitative efforts.

Pelvic Fractures

Pelvic ring fractures are uncommon in children, but they rank second to head injury in terms of complications, particularly life-threatening visceral injuries.[29] Associated injuries occur in 67%, with long-term morbidity in 30%.[29] Unstable pelvic fractures increase the potential for blood loss and, as with the adult, external fixation may be necessary.[30]

Chest Injury

In the study by Nakayama and associates[31] of chest injuries in children, 97% of the injuries were caused by blunt trauma. These researchers noted an associated head, abdominal, or orthopaedic injury in 68%. Significant intrathoracic injuries can occur without rib fractures in 52%.[31] Because the soft chest wall in children offers less protection to underlying lung parenchyma and allows direct transfer of energy to the underlying lung, more than 50%

FIGURE 3

Ogden Classification Schematic patterns of injury. This expanded version of a Salter-Harris classification allows classification of more complex variations on epiphyseal injuries. **1A,** Propagation across the physeal cartilage. **1B,** Propagation across the diseased primary spongiosa (e.g., leukemia, thalassemia), with the physeal interface variably involved. **1C,** Disruption of a localized segment of the physis. **2A,** Partial propagation across both the physis and metaphysis. **2B,** Free and attached metaphyseal fragments. **2C,** Propagation across both the primary spongiosa and metaphysis. **2D,** Localized disruption of the physis at the point of propagation into the metaphysis. **3A,** Epiphyseal fragment with propagation through the physis. **3B,** Epiphyseal fragment with propagation through the primary spongiosa. **3C,** Crushing injury to peripheral physis. **3D,** Nonarticular cartilage avulsion (e.g., ischial tuberosity). **4A,** Combined epiphyseal-physeal-metaphyseal fragment. **4B,** Epiphyseal-physeal-metaphyseal fragment combined with type 3A or 3B lesion. **4C,** Propagation through a nonarticular epiphyseal region (e.g., intraepiphyseal cartilage of the developing femoral neck). **5,** Longitudinal growth retardation of a major physeal segment. **6,** Avulsion or crushing of the peripheral physis (zone of Ranvier). **7A,** Osteochondral fragment involving the physis of the secondary ossification center. **7B,** Chondral fragment involving hypertrophic cells of the physis of the secondary ossification center. **8,** A metaphyseal fracture temporarily cuts off the nutrient artery (N), causing transient ischemia to the metaphyseal segment between the fracture and the physis. **9,** Damage to periosteum, with or without discrete osseous injury, disrupts normal membranous ossification. (Reproduced with permission from Ogden JA: Skeletal growth mechanism injury pattern. *J Pediatr Orthop* 1982;2:371–377.)

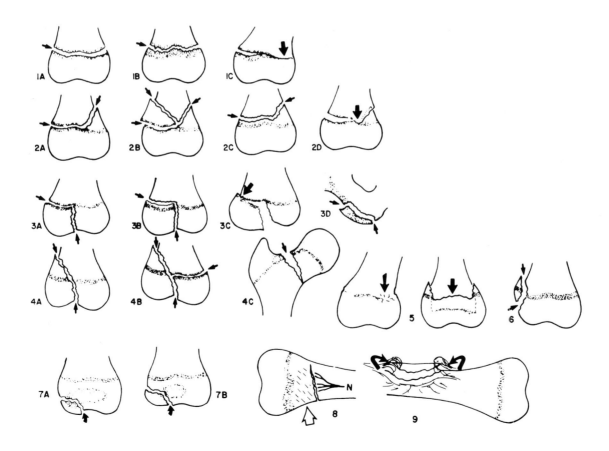

ot children with chest injuries sustain a pulmonary contusion. There is a relatively high incidence of pneumothorax (37%) and tension pneumothorax (23%).[31]

Arterial Injuries

Most vascular injuries in children are caused by penetrating trauma, and only 18% are associated with fracture, usually from motor vehicle accidents and falls.[32] Typically, the artery involved is near the fracture. For example, injury to the common femoral artery is often associated with intertrochanteric hip fractures and hip dislocation, whereas superficial femoral and profunda femoral injuries occur with subtrochanteric and midshaft femoral fractures. Injuries to the vessels about the knee are associated with fractures of the distal femoral epiphysis and proximal tibial epiphysis or with knee dislocation.[33-35] A skeletal injury in the proximity of a major vessel with a pulse deficit is highly suggestive of vascular injury.[36] If the pulse does not return following reduction of the fracture or dislocation, arteriographic evaluation should be obtained. Arterial spasm is common in children.[37,38] Trauma to the intima with late development of thrombosis should be suspected if pulses are initially palpable and then disappear, particularly with injuries about the knee.[34,39] Frequently, there is good capillary flow, because the amount of blood flow required to maintain viability of the skin and subcutaneous structures is much less than that required by muscle.[34]

In adults, the limb salvage rate is 90% if circulation is established within six hours. After eight hours, the amputation rate climbs to 72% to 90%.[34,39] Stanford and associates[32] found that the tissues of a child's limb, particularly the nerves and muscles, are less able to survive prolonged periods of ischemia. Thus, in children, a delay greater than six hours was associated with a poor result in 77%.[32] With massive crush injuries and collateral vessel damage, a six-hour period of warm ischemia may be too long.[40] The indications for fasciotomies in children are the same as in an adult, but fasciotomy should not include fibulectomy, which can lead to valgus angulation and long-term deformity of the ankle.[33,34]

TABLE 5
Severity classification for open fractures

Grade	Description
I	Wound < 1 cm
II	Transitional wound (1–10 cm)
III	Wound > 10 cm
IIIA	Extensive soft-tissue injury
IIIB	Reconstructive soft tissue
IIIC	Vascular injury

Initial bony fixation provides maximum skeletal stability and reduces further trauma to the soft tissue, nerves, and collateral blood vessels. Ideally, fracture fixation should precede vascular repair, because vascular repair is easier following good fracture stabilization.[33] However, revascularization cannot be delayed when limb ischemia is approaching six hours. In selected cases, indwelling arterial and venous shunts can be very beneficial in reducing the risk of compartment syndrome during the time required to stabilize the fracture.[4,21,33] In the severely traumatized limb, external fixation can shorten surgical time. However, if time permits and soft-tissue coverage can be achieved, internal fixation is preferable. Similarly, surgical repair of nerve lacerations is facilitated with bony stabilization, and 45% of nerve injuries are associated with fracture and arterial injury.[35]

INDICATIONS FOR FRACTURE STABILIZATION

The most common indications for fixation are displaced epiphyseal fractures (Salter-Harris types III and IV), displaced intra-articular fractures, unstable fractures, fractures in the multiply injured child, and fractures associated with extensive loss of muscle and soft tissue.[22,23,28,30,41,42] Children with a Modified Injury Severity Scale of 3 or 4 and a concomitant chest or abdominal injury should have fractures stabilized. Surgical reduction of fractures in the child is often required with head injury, burns, vascular injury, floating knee, and severe soft-tissue injuries (lawn mower or propeller injuries).[14,23,28,40] Avulsion fractures of the tibial tubercle require open reduction and internal fixation to resist displacement by the strong pull of the quadriceps.[23,41] Femur fractures should not be treated with tibial traction if there is a serious ligamentous injury to the knee. Ligamentous injuries about the knee appear to be increasing in frequency, and recognition and reconstruction are improved if the fractures are stabilized.[43] In general, the older child or adolescent should be treated as an adult and the fractures stabilized to avoid the complications associated with prolonged traction and/or cast immobilization.[40]

In children, as with adults, rapid and immediate fracture stabilization reduces the need for ventilatory support, time in the intensive care unit, and hospital stay.[12,13] Children undergoing immediate surgical stabilization have fewer complications than those stabilized after three days.[12,13] Fracture fixation facilitates wound care, provides soft-tissue stabilization, and preserves vascularity to the bone (both endosteal and periosteal) and soft tissue. By restoring and maintaining normal extremity growth and function, it is possible to prevent major complications such as premature epiphyseal closure and malunion.[22,42]

As the child ages and approaches adolescence, one must be aware of osseous maturation.[11] The bones are approaching their adult configuration and, although there may be remaining epiphyseal growth, they have less potential for remodeling even minor variations in angulation. There is limited ability to remodel rotation abnormalities at any age. This transition from adolescence to adulthood can be extremely variable, and further assessment of bone age can be easily obtained with a hand and wrist test for bone age.

Bohn and Durbin[28] recently called attention to the problem of the floating knee or ipsilateral fracture of the femur and tibia. In general, patients younger than 10 years of age who have this injury respond well to closed treatment,

femoral traction (90/90) and short leg cast followed by a hip spica.[28] However, in older children and adolescents whose femoral fractures were treated with traction, there was an increased incidence of complications (40%), including malunion-nonunion, angulation, or refracture.[28] In this group, surgical stabilization of the femoral fracture was associated with fewer complications and better results. Importantly, the incidence of tibial complications in this older group was 50%, even in those treated with open reduction or external fixation.[28] The tibial problems may be related to greater injury severity rather than age.

All patients with ipsilateral fracture of the femur and tibia should be evaluated carefully for a ligamentous injury to the knee. Where possible, stress roentgenograms should be a part of the examination. In the young child, this evaluation may be done after the distal femoral traction pin has been placed. If the knee ligaments are injured and require repair, stabilization of the fractures will facilitate their repair and permit early knee motion. The inability to achieve or maintain a satisfactory closed reduction of the tibial fracture and open fractures that are associated with severe soft-tissue injuries are indications for operative stabilization of the tibial fractures. This is true for patients of any age.[28]

BONE FIXATION

Internal Fixation

It is preferable to traverse the epiphysis with smooth pins and avoid the epiphyseal plate. However, crossing the growth plate can be tolerated in certain circumstances if the pins are smooth and are placed close to the anatomic center of the epiphysis. Threaded pins and those that pass close to the margin of the growth plate are more often associated with bridging and growth disturbance. Creative solutions, such as fixing the Thurston-Holland fragment in type II injuries or fixation of both fragments in the type IV, can be used.[22] In Thompson and associates'[42] study of internal fixation of children's fractures, complication rates were higher than expected (18% in preteens and 12% in adolescents), but were minor. All attempts should be made to save as much periosteum as possible. Often, the periosteal tube can be salvaged and considerable new bone formation can occur from it and from the surrounding soft-tissue after injury.

In the adolescent, the size and structure of the bone is nearly adult, and the same techniques and equipment can be used as are used for adults. Intramedullary rods for femoral fractures and screws for hip fractures are good examples. In younger children, it is necessary to modify techniques and equipment used in order to accommodate their small size and to avoid interruption of growth. In children, internal fixation is preferable to external fixation. Internal fixation in nonarticular fractures in children does not have to be perfect.[29] Small flexible rods and short flexible plates can be used as temporary measures, because the bone heals very quickly, and many children can be later be immobilized in casts to supplement the fixation after associated injuries have been treated.[23,44,45]

With internal fixation it is important to retrieve the implant as soon as healing of the fracture permits. Fixation devices can act as stress risers and can lead to refracture. These devices can also be stress shielding, which will inhibit normal bone remodeling and appositional growth in the young child. They can also provide a focus for late infection.

External Fixation

These devices are primarily used for children who have open fractures with significant skin loss or burns, and for those who cannot be treated by internal fixation for whatever reason.[30,46] External fixation is helpful for children with polytrauma and multiple fractures, for those requiring fasciotomy, or for treating extensive contaminated fractures that require that the wound be left open.[46] In situations where there is extensive bone loss, limb length can be maintained during the initial period of debridement and/or until satisfactory skin coverage is achieved.[23] The limb can be transferred to a cast when skin coverage is satisfactory and early fracture stability is present.[46]

The fixators may be left in place for 7 to 10 weeks.[30,46] Meticulous daily pin care is required. Placing the large half-pins creates considerable heat in the bone, which can cause necrosis (ring sequestrum). Twenty to 50% of the children have drainage from their pin sites but, fortunately, few develop chronic osteomyelitis (2%).[26,46] The epiphyseal plate should be avoided, because pin tract infection or the heat from insertion can injure the growth plate. However, in unusual circumstances, the epiphysis can be used for external fixation if the pins are small and carefully placed. The pins may cause a reaction that stimulates more growth than is seen when conventional traction/cast treatments are used.[26,46] Healing is delayed in open fractures, requiring an average of five months compared with 3.3 months for closed fractures.[26] The time to union is related to the soft-tissue injury, type of fracture, amount of segmental bone loss, and occurrence of infection. Refracture after removal of the fixator must be guarded against.[26] Reff[30] recommends large diameter half pins (4 to 5 mm), wide skin incisions around the pin entry sites, meticulous pin care, and dynamization across the fracture afterwards to stimulate complete healing. In his series, following these recommendations significantly reduced the incidence of complications.[30] Decreased joint range of motion was noted.[30]

THE HIP AND ACETABULUM

FRACTURES OF THE HIP

Fractures of the hip and acetabulum are rare in children; fewer than 1% of all hip fractures occur in children or adolescents.[47] Serious complications, however, are reported to occur in as many as 60% of children with these fractures,[47-56] which makes accurate diagnosis and appropriate treatment especially important.

Anatomy

Most of the complications associated with hip and acetabular fractures in children are influenced by the growth and developmental patterns of the hip and the changing blood supply of the proximal femoral epiphysis. At birth, a single physis is present in the proximal femur. Between the ages of 6 and 12 months, this separates into two centers of ossification (Fig. 4).[57] The ossific nucleus of the greater trochanter appears at approximately 4 years of age in both boys and girls.

The high incidence of osteonecrosis after hip fractures is related to the blood supply of the femur, as observed by Trueta,[58] Chung,[59] and Ogden.[60] Their findings are summarized as follows:

(1) The vessels of the ligamentum teres are of little importance and contribute a small percentage of the blood supply to the femoral head until the age of 8 years; in adults, they contribute only 20%.

(2) At birth, the predominant blood supply to the femoral head is from the branches of the medial and lateral circumflex arteries that traverse the femoral neck. As the physis develops, it prevents these vessels from penetrating into the femoral head, so that by the age of 4 years this metaphyseal blood supply is virtually nonexistent.

(3) As the metaphyseal vessels diminish, the lateral epiphyseal vessels become dominant and become the primary supply of the femoral head as they bypass the physeal barrier. Ogden[60] noted that capsulotomy of the hip will not damage the blood supply of the femoral head unless it violates the intertrochanteric notch or damages the posteroinferior or posterosuperior vessels along the femoral neck.

(4) By the age of 4 years, the lateral posterosuperior vessels predominate and supply all the anterolateral portion of the proximal femoral epiphysis. The posteroinferior and posterosuperior arteries persist through life as the blood supply to the femoral head.

Mechanism of injury

In contrast to adult hip fractures, most hip fractures in children are caused by severe trauma. With the exception of the proximal femoral physis, the femoral neck in children is extremely strong, and high-velocity forces, such as falls from heights and accidents involving moving vehicles, are necessary to cause fractures.

Occasionally, fractures can be caused by other trauma, as in child abuse, or by pathologic conditions, such as unicameral bone cyst or fibrous dysplasia.

Classification

Children's hip fractures generally are classified according to the system outlined by Delbet and modified by others (Fig. 5):[49,50] Type 1, transepiphyseal separation, with or without dislocation of the femoral head from the acetabulum; type 2, transcervical fracture, displaced or nondisplaced; type 3, cervicotrochanteric fracture, displaced or nondisplaced; and type 4, intertrochanteric fracture.

Examination and Radiographic Evaluation

Type 1 (transepiphyseal separation) injuries (Fig. 6) assume several different patterns, depending on the age of the patient and the presence of such conditions as metabolic or neoplastic disease. Neonatal epiphysiolysis is uncommon, but can occur during birth trauma; it generally is treated closed and has a relatively low incidence of osteonecrosis. In some cases, the diagnosis must be made by arthrography, because in infants radiographs generally show only upward and lateral displacement of the femoral shaft.

Differential diagnoses in adolescents include acute or chronic slipped capital femoral epiphysis. Clinical symptoms of this injury are characteristic: Swelling in the inguinal crease, gluteal area, and proximal thigh; holding of the limb in external rotation, flexion, and adduction; resistance to any movement; pain and, often, crepitation with hip motion; and pseudoparalysis of the affected limb in infants.

Types 2, 3, and 4 fractures are much more common than are type 1 fractures. The history is one of severe trauma, followed by sudden pain in the hip and an inability to stand or walk. The injured extremity is held in external rotation and slight adduction and may be flexed to relieve capsular distension. Active hip motion is impossible if the fracture is displaced, and passive motion, especially flexion, abduction, and internal rotation, is markedly restricted and painful. The extremity may be shortened as much as 1 to 2 cm. Anteroposterior and lateral radiographs will confirm the

FIGURE 4
Transformation of a single physis into separate physes for the femoral head and greater trochanter. From left to right: Newborn, 4 months, 1 year, 4 years, and 6 years. (Reproduced with permission from Edgren W: Coxa plana: A clinical and radiological investigation with particular reference to the importance of the metaphyseal changes for the final shape of the proximal part of the femur. *Acta Orthop Scand* 1965;84(suppl):1–129.)

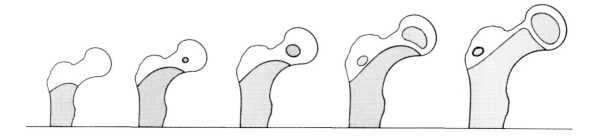

FIGURE 5
Classification of hip fractures in children. **Left**, Type 1-transepiphyseal. **Center left**, Type 2-transcervical. **Center right**, Type 3-cervicotrochanteric. **Right**, Type 4-intertrochanteric (Reproduced with permission from Swiontkowski MF, Winquist RA: Displaced hip fractures in children and adolescents. *J Trauma* 1986;26:384–388.)

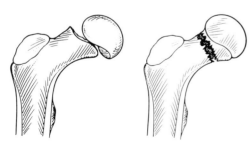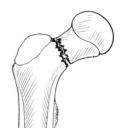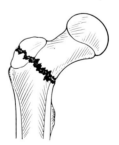

clinical impression (Fig. 7). The radiographs should be studied to determine the direction of the fracture line, the degree of angulation, and the amount of posterior tilt, and to detect the rare displacement of the femoral head from its normal location in the acetabulum.

Treatment Guidelines

Commonly accepted treatment recommendations are given in Outline 1.

Timing of Treatment

As a general rule, fractures of the hip in children do not require emergency treatment but should be treated as promptly as possible. Type 1 fractures with dislocations of the femoral head, however, do require immediate treatment. If surgery is required for any type of hip fracture, it should be performed within 24 hours of injury if possible. Although some authors have recommended immediate treat-

FIGURE 6
Type 1 fracture (transepiphyseal
separation) of left hip in a 5-year-old girl.

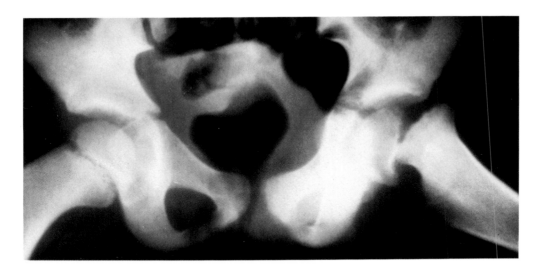

ment to reduce the incidence of osteone-crosis, the literature does not clearly indicate that the timing of treatment has an effect on the development of this problem.

Surgical Treatment

Children younger than 6 years of age can be placed on an image table. For children aged 7 years and older, a standard fracture table can be used. A straight lateral trochanteric approach is used if a satisfactory closed reduction is obtained. The reduction maneuver usually consists of traction and slight internal rotation. An unacceptable reduction is indicated by a varus position or excessive displacement on the anteroposterior or lateral radiographs, as determined by comparison views of the opposite hip. Although the exact degree of displacement considered unacceptable is not clearly defined, a general rule is that no displacement exceeding 10% or 20% of the width of the femoral neck should be accepted, because further varus angulation is likely. Image intensification is used to check the reduction and to aid in the placement of guide wires and cannulated screws or other fixation devices. Cast immobilization in a spica cast

usually is recommended for children up to 10 or 11 years of age.

Generalized statements follow concerning types of pins, number of pins, length of cast immobilization, or even the necessity of cast immobilization. Each of these factors depends on the age of the patient and the type of hip fracture. For most fractures in children younger than 6 years of age, two cannulated mini or small-fragment hip screws are preferable for femoral neck fractures. Fractures in children aged 7 to 12 years may be fixed with two or three cannulated hip screws, depending on the size of the femoral neck and the size of the screws. Usually types 1, 2, or 3 fractures can be stabilized with cannulated screws; type 4 fractures may require fixation with a hip compression screw device with a sideplate. Fractures in children aged 13 years or older usually can be treated with multiple pin fixation or a hip compression screw as in adults.

If possible, cannulated screws should not cross the proximal femoral physis unless the fracture cannot be stabilized without doing so. Stable fixation of type 3 (cervicotrochanteric) fractures and some type 2 (transcervical) frac-

FIGURE 7
Top, Displaced type 2 (transcervical) fracture of right hip in 15-year-old boy.
Bottom, Treated by closed reduction and fixation with two cannulated screws.

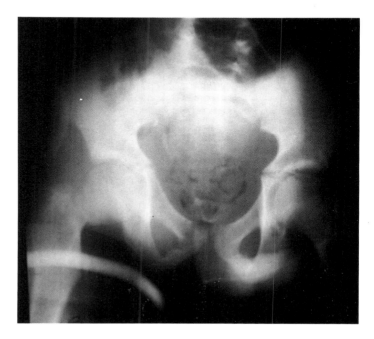

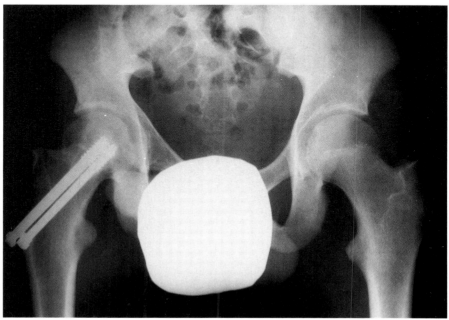

FIGURE 8
Nondisplaced type 3 (cervicotrochanteric) fracture in 5-year-old boy treated in abduction spica cast.

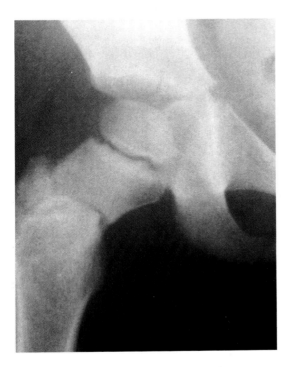

tures usually is possible without crossing the physis (Figs. 8 and 9); however, type 1 fractures require pin fixation crossing the physis into the femoral head. Some authors have reported that smooth pin fixation is preferable to threaded pins for these fractures,[50] but threaded pins usually are used.

Type 4 fractures in children aged 6 years or younger, except in patients with multiple injuries or burns, may be reduced with three to six weeks of skeletal traction and then immobilized in a hip abduction cast for a total treatment period of 12 weeks. Fractures in older children (aged 7 to 12 years) often cannot be satisfactorily reduced with traction, and open reduction and internal fixation with a pediatric hip screw may be required; a hip spica cast is used for eight to 12 weeks after surgery, depending on the stability of fixation. As children approach the teenage years, during the final years of skeletal growth, type 4 fractures may be treated as in adults with a hip compression screw and sideplate device that crosses the physis into the femoral head, and no postoperative immobilization (Fig. 10).

Surgical Alternatives

If satisfactory closed reduction can be obtained but not maintained, the use of percutaneous pins inserted through multiple small incisions, with image intensification control,

OUTLINE 1
Treatment guidelines for hip fractures in children

Type 1	Transepiphyseal separation
	Without dislocation—gentle closed reduction and pin fixation
	With dislocation—attempted gentle closed reduction; if not successful, immediate open reduction and pin fixation
Type 2	Transcervical fracture—closed or open reduction and pin fixation for both displaced and nondisplaced fractures
Type 3	Cervicotrochanteric fracture
	Displaced—gentle closed reduction or open reduction and pin fixation
	Nondisplaced—abduction spica cast (Fig. 5)
Type 4	Skeletal traction followed by hip abduction spica cast for 12 weeks or open reduction for unsuccessful reduction in juveniles or older adolescents

FIGURE 9
Left, Displaced type 3 (cervicotrochanteric) fracture in 5-year-old girl. **Right**, After reduction and fixation with cannulated, minifragment screws that do not cross the physis.

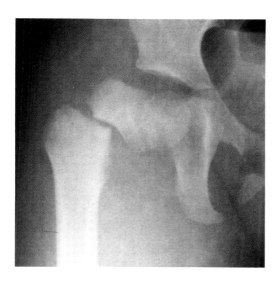

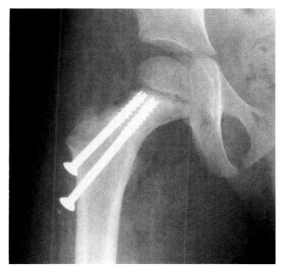

may be indicated. Knowles pins or similar devices may be used if cannulated screws are not available. A hip abduction spica cast is used for postoperative immobilization. If an acceptable closed reduction cannot be obtained, open reduction through a Watson-Jones approach occasionally may be required for femoral neck fractures, followed by pin fixation. No absolute time limit for removal of the hardware has been established. In general, fixation devices are removed in skeletally immature patients within 12 to 18 months of injury, if the fracture has healed, to prevent bony overgrowth.

Complications

The ideal result after hip fractures in children is union of the fracture without osteonecrosis or growth disturbance of the capital femoral physis. Unfortunately, complications are frequent.

Osteonecrosis is the most common, and most devastating, sequela of hip fractures in chil-

dren. It occurs in approximately 42% of children with hip fractures and is usually evident within 9 to 12 months after injury (Fig. 11). Osteonecrosis is most common after type 1 fractures, with a reported incidence approaching 100%.[47,48,52,55] It occurs in about 52% of patients with type 2 fractures, in 27% of those with type 3 fractures, and in 14% of those with type 4 fractures.[48] Ratliff[47] described three patterns of osteonecrosis after hip fractures in children (Fig. 12). In type 1 there is diffuse increased density and sclerosis, accompanied by total involvement and complete collapse of the femoral head; in type 2 there is increased density localized to a portion of the epiphysis and accompanied by minimal collapse of the femoral head; and in type 3 there is increased sclerosis of the femoral neck from the fracture line to the physis, but sparing the femoral head.

Nonunion occurs in 5% to 8% of fractures,[47,48,53-55] an incidence similar to that in adult hip fractures. Closed treatment, espe-

FIGURE 10
Top, Type 4 (intertrochanteric) fracture in 14-year-old boy with unicameral bone cyst. **Bottom,** After open reduction, curettage, grafting, and internal fixation with hip compression screw.

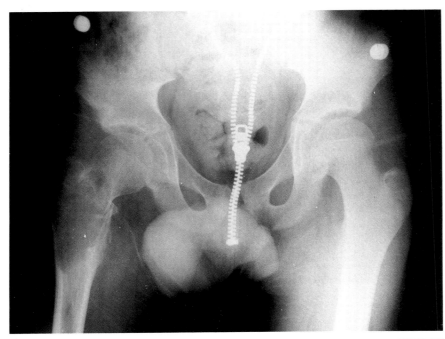

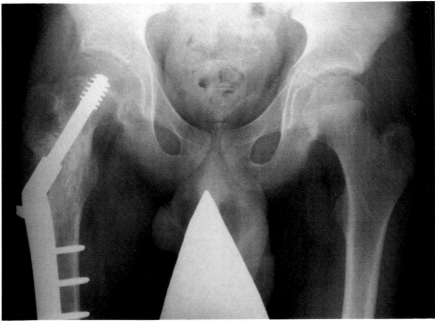

cially of types 2 and 3 fractures, is associated with increased incidences of nonunion and coxa vara. Internal fixation after acceptable reduction decreases the incidence of nonunion because it does not allow varus angulation or late displacement. If nonunion or severe coxa vara deformity after fracture union (Fig. 13) requires surgery, subtrochanteric valgus osteotomy can give excellent long-term results if osteonecrosis is not present.

Premature closure of the physis, in the absence of osteonecrosis, generally results in only minimal leg-length inequality in older children, because the proximal femoral physis contributes approximately 1/8 inch per year of growth in the femur. A combination of osteonecrosis and premature physeal closure, however, can result in significant discrepancies. All children with premature physeal closure should be followed with yearly scanograms and radiographs of the hand and wrist to determine bone age, and the results of this testing should be plotted on the Moseley growth prediction chart. Any leg-length inequality after premature physeal closure is moderately progressive rather than static, and long-term treatment, including a well-timed epiphysiodesis in most patients, should be carefully considered. The younger the child at the time of fracture and the greater the growth potential of the proximal femoral physis, the more the risk of growth disturbance, especially if osteonecrosis occurs or if the physis has been crossed by fracture fixation. In rare cases, symptomatic trochanteric overgrowth in children older than 8 years can require trochanteric transfer.

FRACTURES OF THE ACETABULUM

Anatomy

The pelvis is formed from three primary centers of ossification; the ischium, the pubis, and the ilium. The epiphyses of the three bones meet as the triradiate cartilage, which allows integrated development of the pelvic bones and enlargement of the hemispheric acetabulum (Fig. 14). Any injury that causes premature fusion of the triradiate cartilage can

FIGURE 11
Osteonecrosis three years after type 1 (transepiphyseal) fracture.

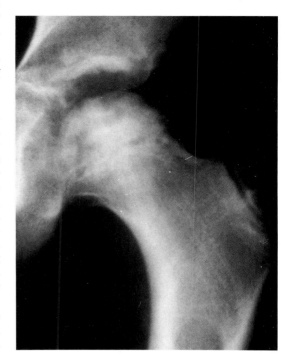

cause thickening of the medial acetabular wall and a shallow acetabulum, leading to progressive subluxation of the femoral head.

Incidence and Classification

Fractures of the acetabulum occur in approximately 10% of children with pelvic fractures.[61-63] These are of four types (Outline 2). Type A (small fragment) fractures usually involve the posterior rim of the acetabulum (Fig. 15), because posterior hip dislocation is approximately ten times more common than anterior dislocation. Type B (large, stable linear) fractures are associated with pelvic fractures that cause compression of the pelvis and a break in the pelvic ring with fracture into the acetabulum (Fig. 16); these may involve the triradiate cartilage. Type C (linear) fractures with instability of the hip joint usually occur when forces are transmitted along the femoral neck, causing a large fracture of the superior

FIGURE 12
Three types of osteonecrosis of femoral head (from left to right, types 1, 2, and 3). (Reproduced with permission from Ratliff AHC: *J Bone Joint Surg* 1962;44B:528.)

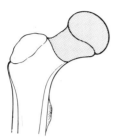 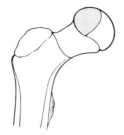 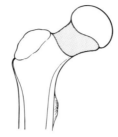

FIGURE 13
Coxa vara deformity after angulated type 3 (cervicotrochanteric) fracture treated with spica cast.

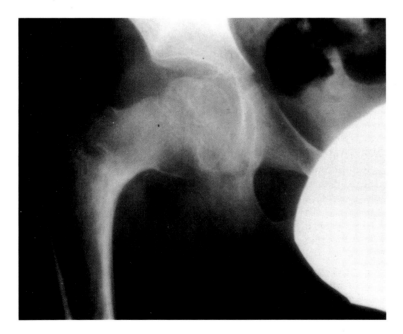

dome of the acetabulum and subluxation or dislocation of the femoral head; these are similar to comparable acetabular fractures in adults, but in children they may also involve the triradiate cartilage. Type D fractures, with central fracture-dislocation of the hip (Fig. 17), generally occur when forces are transmitted through the femoral neck into the ace-

FIGURE 14

Epiphyses of ischium, pubis, and ilium meet to form the triradiate cartilage.

(Reproduced with permission from Scuderi G, Bronson MJ: Triradiate cartilage injury: Report of two cases and review of the literature. *Clin Orthop* 1987;217:179–189.)

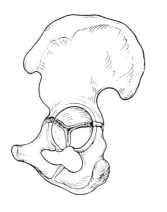 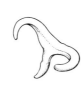

OUTLINE 2
Classification of acetabular fractures

A	Avulsion of a small fragment that most often occurs with hip dislocation
B	Undisplaced, stable linear fracture that occurs with other pelvic fractures
C	Linear fracture with hip joint instability
D	Fracture secondary to central fracture-dislocation of the acetabulum

should be remembered, however, that purely cartilaginous damage is not revealed by computed tomography, but it may be visible on arthrogram or MRI.

tabulum. In growing children, this injury can cause gross disruption of the triradiate cartilage. A variant of the central fracture-dislocation is a medially displaced fracture of the ischium and acetabulum that is known as Walther's fracture.

Examination and Radiographic Evaluation

Because most acetabular fractures occur in association with other, more severe injuries, isolated symptoms of acetabular injury often cannot be determined.

Standard radiographic views of the pelvis may not adequately demonstrate acetabular fracture configurations. Tilt, oblique, and Judet views may help determine the amount of displacement. Comparison views of the opposite hip also may be helpful. Computed tomographic scanning is more sensitive than plain radiography in detecting acetabular fractures,[48] especially of the acetabular roof and posterior wall, and can help determine the size and stability of fracture fragments, can make fracture classification easier, and can identify associated soft-tissue injuries. It

Treatment

The goal of treatment of acetabular fractures in children is restoration of joint congruity and hip stability. In addition, in growing children anatomic alignment of a severely displaced triradiate cartilage fracture should be attempted to prevent growth disturbance that would result in a shallow, dysplastic acetabulum. Injuries to the triradiate cartilage in children require special attention. Although isolated injury to the triradiate cartilage is rare, it appears that the most significant factor in the development of acetabular dysplasia is the age of the child at the time of injury.[48,62,64,65] According to Bucholz and associates,[61] children younger than 10 years of age are especially at risk (Fig. 18). According to reports in the literature, the average age at time of injury in children who develop acetabular dysplasia after triradiate cartilage injury is 7 years. Any child with injury to the triradiate cartilage should be examined annually until skeletal maturity, and any significant acetabular dysplasia should be treated by appropriate pelvic or femoral osteotomies.

FIGURE 15
Type A (small fragment) acetabular fracture
in 16-year-old girl with traumatic hip
dislocation.

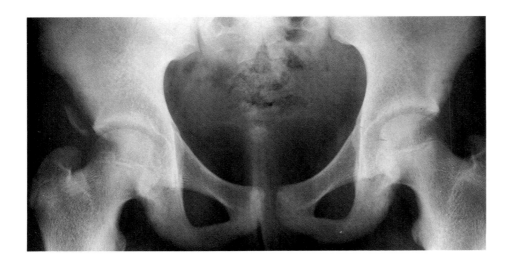

FIGURE 16
Type B (large, linear, stable) acetabular
fracture (on right) in 4-year-old girl.

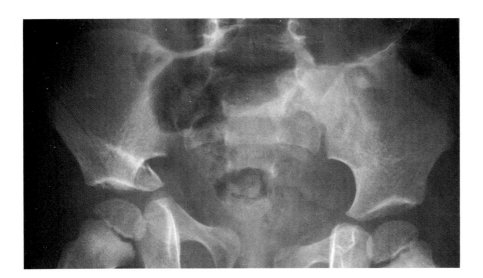

FIGURE 17
FIGURE 17
Top left, Type D acetabular fracture with central fracture-dislocation of the hip.
Bottom left, Five years after injury. **Right**, At long-term follow-up, osteonecrosis and degenerative joint disease are evident.

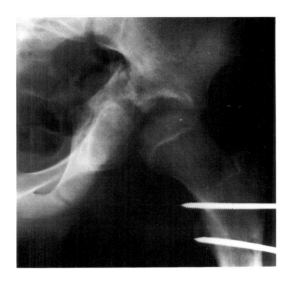

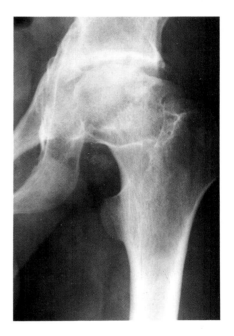

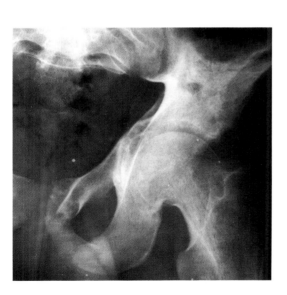

Small fragment (type A) fractures can be treated by a short period of bed rest, followed by early ambulation when symptoms subside.

If hip dislocation occurred, radiographs, computed tomographic scans, or arthrograms after reduction should be carefully examined to de-

FIGURE 18

Premature closure of the triradiate cartilage (**left**), results in proliferation of articular cartilage, thickening of acetabular floor, and dysplasic acetabulum with subluxation of femoral head (**right**). (Reproduced with permission from Scuderi G, Bronson MJ: Triradiate cartilage injury: Report of two cases and review of the literature. *Clin Orthop* 1987;217:179–189.)

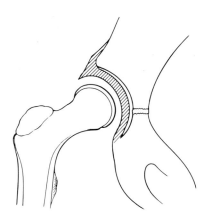 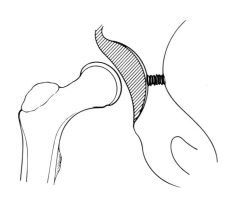

tect any joint incongruity caused by bony or cartilaginous fragments or an inverted labrum in the acetabulum. Open reduction is indicated only for fractures in which fragments displaced into the joint cause a nonconcentric hip reduction.

Nondisplaced linear (type B) fractures should be treated as pelvic fractures, with stability determined by other breaks in the pelvic ring. Unstable pelvic fractures may require external fixation, traction, or a combination of external and internal fixation, as in adults. If there are no other fractures of the pelvic ring, displacement of the acetabular fracture should be prevented by the use of longitudinal traction until the fracture unites. This may require three to six weeks in traction and an additional four to six weeks of crutch use.

Large displaced fractures of the acetabular roof (type C) in adolescents should be treated as in adults. Anatomic congruity of the acetabular fragments and stability of the hip joint are the goals of treatment. If these can be accomplished by skeletal traction, this is continued for eight to 16 weeks for children younger than 10 years old. Open reduction may be required if traction does not achieve congruity and stability, as determined by repeat radiographs and computed tomography scans. An extensile approach, including anterior and posterior dissection, may be necessary for reduction, and multiple internal fixation techniques, including plate and screw fixation, may be required to maintain the reduction in adolescent patients with large acetabular fragments, minimal comminution, and an incongruous reduction.

Central-fracture dislocations and Walther's fractures (type D) have been reported to have poor results regardless of the type of treatment. The aim of treatment is to reduce the forces of the femoral head on the acetabulum by the application of distal and lateral traction. Distal traction is applied first and the reduction is checked on radiographs. If alignment is not acceptable, lateral traction is applied through threaded pins in the trochanteric and, if necessary, cervical hip region. The amount of traction and time in traction depend on the age and size of the child. Reports indicate that adults who were treated with 12 to 16 weeks of traction and who were nonweightbearing for three to six months had better clinical results than those who were allowed early weightbearing. The results of severe central fracture-dislocations appear to be poor in children, and surgical intervention should probably be avoided, because the possible complications of such extensive surgery will not better the chances for a satisfactory result.

FEMUR FRACTURES IN CHILDREN

Femoral shaft fractures are one of the most common major orthopaedic injuries in children and adolescents. While most femur fractures can be successfully treated by conservative methods (skin or skeletal traction, casting),[66] many centers are now electing to use surgery to treat such fractures, for reasons of cost, for psychological considerations, and to avoid long periods of immobilization.[40,44,45]

ANATOMY

Because the femoral shaft is of a consistently tubular shape, with moderate metaphyseal flaring distally, fracture patterns are consistent throughout the length of the bone. A thick cuff of thigh muscles surrounds the bone, making neurovascular injuries rare. The distal femoral physis is increasingly susceptible to growth arrest as it matures and becomes convoluted with mamillary processes; it can suffer unrecognized injury at the time of the femur fracture, or during skeletal pin insertion or internal fixation.[67]

Most femur fractures easily reduce with longitudinal traction. In fractures of the subtrochanteric region (above the insertion of the gluteus maximus), the proximal fragment flexes and abducts, and special reduction techniques may be required to bring the distal fragment into alignment.

The femoral periosteum is thick and highly osteogenic until physeal closure. Periosteal new bone formation in children can be dramatic, filling in large bone defects without bone grafting (Fig. 19). The periosteum also tends to remain adequately intact to control rotation of the fragments, making rotational malalignment of childhood femur fractures rare, regardless of treatment method.[68]

REMODELING AND OVERGROWTH

In rapidly growing children, residual angular deformities following femur fracture have a strong tendency to remodel. Depending on the age of the child, deformities of 30 degrees in the sagittal plane and 20 degrees in the frontal plane are acceptable.

In children aged 2 to 10 years, the femur will generally overgrow by 1 to 2 cm as a result of the hyperemia of injury and repair. Slight overriding of the shaft fragments is desirable in this age group, and overgrowth will continue for 12 to 18 months after injury. Adolescents lose this ability and require restoration of bone length for the best result.

MECHANISM OF INJURY

Femur fractures are generally the result of major injury, as can occur when a bicyclist or pedestrian collides with a motor vehicle. Associated major injuries, including head injury, chest injury, intra-abdominal trauma, and other long bone and physeal fractures, are common and can be life-threatening.

In young children, femur fractures are a common finding in child abuse. There is no fracture configuration that is unique to child abuse, but abuse should be considered in any child younger than 3 years of age who has a femoral shaft fracture.

EVALUATION

Initially, femur fractures should be splinted and the patient should be rapidly and thoroughly evaluated for head, chest, intra-abdominal, pelvic, and neurovascular injury. If the patient can cooperate, the evaluation should include testing for tenderness at the knee physes.

In addition to standard anteroposterior and lateral radiographs, all children with a fractured femur should have a film of the pelvis to rule out pelvic or acetabular fractures. Radiographs of the knee, particularly in older children and adolescents, may detect occult fracture of the physes of the distal femur or proximal tibia. Suspected victims of child abuse should have a skeletal series (and, in some cases, a bone scan) to detect other signs of skeletal trauma.

NONSURGICAL TREATMENT

Nonsurgical treatment methods include immediate spica casting, skin traction, and vari-

FIGURE 19

Left, A 12-year-old girl suffered segmental loss of distal femoral shaft after injury with a deer rifle. She was treated by debridement and external fixation; the wound was left open and no bone graft was used. **Center**, Eight weeks later, the segmental loss has filled in with periosteal new bone; the femur is in slight varus. **Right**, One year later, lateral staples were used to correct varus alignment. Note the remodeling of fracture site.

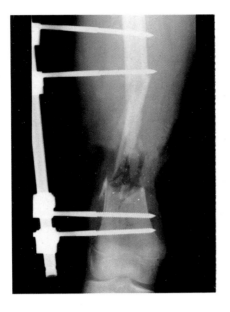 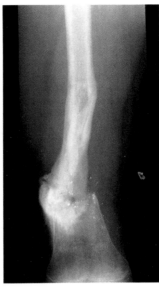 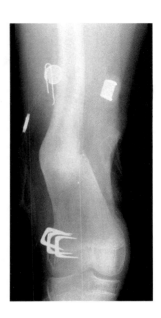

eties of skeletal traction. Each method has its proponents, and none is inherently superior to the others. Goals of nonsurgical treatment should be: union with acceptable length and angulation, avoidance of injury to the physes, and minimization of both hospitalization and social impact of the fracture on the patient and family.

Immediate Spica Casting

Children younger than 2 years of age are treated by immediate application of a double spica cast in a comfortable position; in infants, a "human" position can be used, corresponding to physiologic flexion posturing. Moderate abduction relaxes the iliotibial band and minimizes late shortening and angulation.

Particularly in children younger than 8 years of age, immediate spica casting with general anesthesia allows rapid immobilization, pain relief, and timely discharge of the patient to home. The cast should be carried to the ankles or feet, and molded well around the pelvis.[69,70] Close follow-up with frequent radiographs is necessary to detect any angulation or excessive shortening that might occur, and to allow timely correction, such as cast wedging or reinstitution of traction. However, despite postreduction radiographs that indicate otherwise, some shortening always occurs, but it usually will be made up by overgrowth. Those children with more than 2.5 cm of shortening probably should be considered for traction treatment. Immediate casting may be inappropriate when closed abdominal or pelvic injury is suspected.

Traction

Skin traction is an excellent method for maintaining alignment and comfort while observation (e.g., for abdominal injury) continues.[71] For safety, it is usually inadvisable to attempt to achieve full reduction of length with skin traction; for most children, 5 pounds of traction will achieve acceptable alignment, because overgrowth is expected. Once the child is stable, a double spica cast can be applied over the skin traction and the child can be discharged to home (Fig. 20). In children younger than 8 to 9 years of age, casting can be done within several days of fracture (see above); in older children, skin or skeletal traction may be used with delayed application of spica cast as outlined immediately below.

Skeletal Traction

Skeletal traction is most useful when traction must be prolonged (after the age of 9 to 10, when overgrowth is unlikely) or when reduction is otherwise impossible (subtrochanteric fracture). The traditional traction device for children is a smooth Kirschner wire (K-wire), because it reduces the chance of physeal injury; however, any traction pin may be used. Smooth pins must be inserted at a right angle to the shaft of the bone, or they will migrate laterally. Proper positioning of the pin is most important to avoid injury to the physis, and radiographs of the pin should be taken after placement.

Opinions differ about the use of femoral or tibial skeletal pins, but whichever is used, the surgeon must be knowledgeable about proper placement to avoid injury to the physis. Longitudinal traction with either a tibial or a femoral pin allows reduction of nearly all femur fractures except proximal (subtrochanteric) fractures. For these, 90–90 traction with a femoral pin will be required, with a suspended short-leg cast to aid in positioning the leg. A tibial pin should not be used for 90–90 traction in children, because it can cause stretching of the cruciate ligaments.[72]

When traction is used in older children to maintain length, it must be continued until callus can be seen on radiograph. Because early callus (2.5 to 3 weeks) is weak and will bend, it is wise to wait approximately a week after the first appearance of callus before applying a spica cast. Thus, for children 10 or older, nearly four weeks of hospitalization may be required before casting.

Cast-Brace

While cast-braces have been used in children, they are often painful and require close supervision. Malunion can be a significant problem in more proximal fractures. Cast-brace use has no advantage over more conventional modes of treatment.

Complications of Closed Management

Skin traction can lead to blisters, usually from slippage of the adhesive straps. This can best be avoided by careful application of straps by the physician and by avoidance of excessive traction weight in an unnecessary attempt to regain full length in younger children.

Skeletal traction pins can injure the physis and cause angular deformities or limb-length inequality. Pins can also lead to superficial infection and even osteomyelitis. Younger children treated in skeletal traction with maintenance of full length may exhibit late overgrowth and limb-length inequality.

The most common complication in older children is malunion, usually caused by premature casting when early (and bendable) callus is thought to be strong enough. The angulation (usually anterior and lateral) that occurs does so in the first week after casting. The callus then becomes rigid enough that it cannot be corrected except by surgical means. In such cases, it is best to observe for 1 to 2 years to allow any potential remodeling to occur.

SURGICAL TREATMENT

Accepted indications for surgical treatment of pediatric femur fractures include open fractures (which require debridement and, possibly, fixation), concomitant severe head injury (where posturing and spasticity can lead to difficulty controlling fragments with traction and to malunion), and fractures in older adolescents (which are treated according to adult guidelines). Traditionally, closed fractures of the femoral shaft have been treated by traction. However, the negative psychological effects of prolonged traction and casting, for both the child and the family, have led to a reassessment of traditional nonsurgical treatment of closed femoral shaft fractures, particularly in the adolescent who may be emotionally labile. Several series have demonstrated that routine surgical treatment of femoral shaft

FIGURE 20
A double spica cast applied over skin traction achieves excellent immobilization and allows early discharge from the hospital. Late overgrowth makes up acute shortening that occurs in a cast.

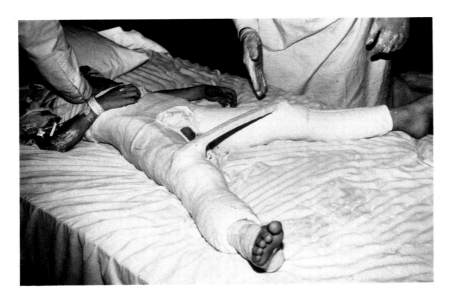

fractures in children as young as 10 years of age can be accomplished safely, with significant reduction in cost, and with the psychological benefit of early return to home and school. Surgical treatment also minimizes malunion, and overgrowth has not been reported as a significant problem in patients 10 years of age and older.[45]

Most orthopaedic surgeons have experience with surgical management of adult femur fractures, and similar techniques can be used (with modification) in the child. A properly equipped operating room and fluoroscopic equipment are mandatory.

Closed Intramedullary Femoral Nailing

Closed intramedullary nailing can be safely done in children as young as 10 to 12 years of age, using conventional techniques. Either lateral or supine positioning is used. It is imperative that surgeons performing intramedullary nailing for children be experienced with the procedure for adults before attempting it in patients who are not skeletally mature.

Prophylactic antibiotics are used. Small implants should be available; some pediatric femurs require a 9 mm nail. The proximal entry site should be kept slightly lateral to the base of the femoral neck. Proximal and distal interlocking are performed for the same indications as in the adult (Fig. 21); it is unnecessary to "dynamize" an interlocked nail, because healing of periosteal new bone is aggressive. Special care should be taken to control distal reaming, and the nail should be left short enough to avoid injuring the distal physis. Leaving the nail slightly prominent facilitates removal, but many children develop heterotopic bone at the tip of the nail, which causes mild pain.

Crutch walking can often begin within 24 hours, with discharge from the hospital 2 to 3 days after surgery. Healing is rapid. Children should be allowed to return to school with crutches as soon as callus is visible on radiograph (1 to 2 weeks).

Routine removal of intramedullary nails in immature patients is appropriate at eight to 12 months after healing is complete.

28

FIGURE 21

Left, Proximal interlocking used in closed intramedullary nailing of femur fracture in an 11-year-old boy. **Right**, The distal end of the rod is kept well proximal to the distal femoral physis. Interlocking can be performed safely at this level under radiographic control.

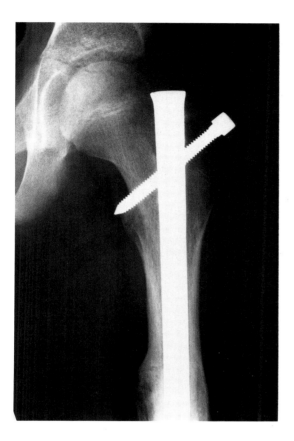
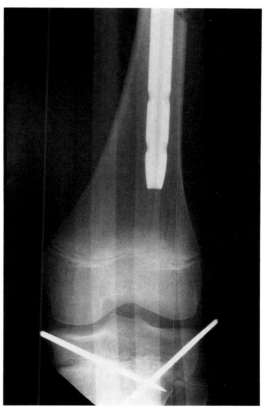

In addition to standard reamed intramedullary nails, flexible nails (such as the Ender nail) can be used, inserting them either antegrade or retrograde. If several nails are used, the fracture is usually rigid enough that casting is unnecessary (Fig. 22).

The special case of intramedullary nailing in young children (under eight to 10 years) for head injury can best be handled by using a small flexible nail (such as a Rush rod). It is inserted laterally through a fenestration distal to the greater trochanter, and the femur is externally immobilized with a spica cast (Fig. 23).

Complications of heterotopic bone and distal physeal injury are noted above. Infection (rare) is best treated by antibiotics and elective reaming, with rod exchange if indicated. Loss of position can be controlled by traction. Nonunion and malunion are extremely rare; overgrowth has not been a problem in reported series. Although arrest of the greater trochanteric apophysis is a theoretical concern, the trochanter grows by appositional bone after age 10, and arrest has not proven to be a problem. Younger children may exhibit some decrease in the thickness of the femoral neck on anteroposterior radiograph. This de-

FIGURE 22

Multiple Ender nails used for internal fixation of a segmental femur fracture in an adolescent. In this case, the pins were inserted antegrade through the greater trochanter; they could also have been inserted retrograde, using radiograph to assure that the distal femoral physis was not violated. No cast fixation was required.

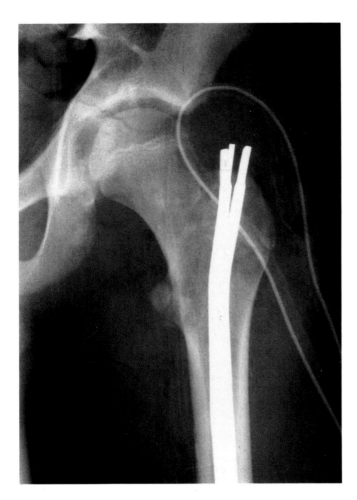
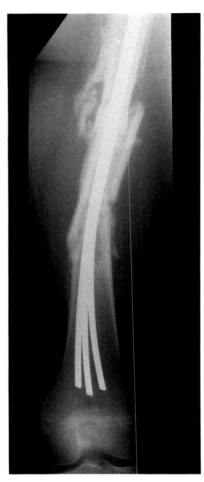

crease, which is of uncertain significance, may represent arrest of the lateral appositional growth of the neck, but no associated long-term problems have been described.

External Fixation

External fixation is used by some surgeons as primary treatment for closed femur fractures in adolescents; it offers no unique advantage over intramedullary nailing, but it can be used if the surgeon prefers. More specific indications for these devices include stabilization of open fractures requiring repeated soft-tissue debridement, and rapid fixation of fractures in unstable multiply-injured children or children with head injuries. External fixators can be used effectively for these indications in children of all ages (not just in those 10 years and up), but overgrowth should be taken into account in younger children.

A rigid single lateral frame (such as the Wagner device) is easiest to use. Often a device designed for the adult humerus is ideally sized for the pediatric femur. The pins can be quickly inserted "blind" by an experienced surgeon in an emergency, with perfect reduction achieved later, using the controls on the device. Fluoroscopy helps achieve optimum placement; the half-pins should penetrate both lateral and medial cortex.

The fixator is left in place until callus is present, at which time it may be removed and the femur protected in a cast. Alternatively, the fixator is adjusted to compress the callus once it has appeared, and weightbearing is allowed.

The complication of pin infection can usually be controlled by antibiotic administration and pin site release or debridement, if necessary. Loss of fixation is treated by reinserting and adjusting the fixator, or by instituting traction (usually skeletal).

The callus that forms with an external fixator is weak and will bend (usually into varus and flexion) if the device is removed too early. This pitfall is similar to that seen in the adolescent treated with skeletal traction (see above). Malunion is avoided by extending the period in the fixator, or by dynamically loading the maturing callus with compression and weightbearing.

Compression Plating

Compression plating is mechanically effective for transverse fractures of the pediatric femur, but it offers few advantages over intramedullary nailing in children older than 10 or 11 years of age. When open fractures with extensive periosteal stripping must be stabilized, plating can be appropriate, because the bone is already exposed and endosteal injury may be avoided. Compression plating also has the advantage of avoiding physeal injury during management of shaft fractures. Generally, only one plate is required in children, rather than two at right angles to each other as used in the adult (Fig. 24). Bone grafting, even for diaphyseal fractures, is unnecessary. Most children undergoing plating should be externally stabilized after surgery with a spica cast.

Compression plates used on the femoral shaft should be electively removed once solid

FIGURE 23
A Rush rod, inserted distal to the greater trochanteric apophysis, can be used in conjunction with a cast for young children with fracture of the femur and severe head injury.

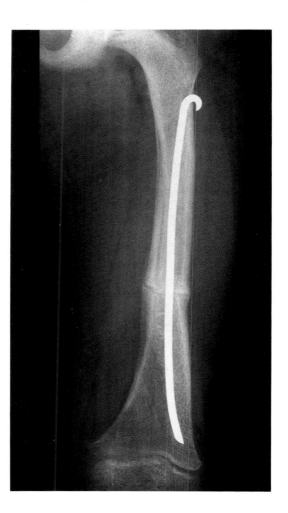

union is achieved. Cast protection (unilateral spica) is often necessary after this procedure.

FRACTURES ABOUT THE KNEE IN CHILDREN

Ligamentous knee injuries, frequently seen in adults, are rare in children.[73] They do occur, however, and stress radiographs are used to

FIGURE 24

Left, A 10-year-old boy hit by a car sustained a fracture to the distal femur. Satisfactory reduction could not be obtained from traction with a proximal tibial pin. **Right**, Open reduction and internal fixation were performed using a plate and screws. The proximal fracture was found to be embedded in the quadriceps mechanism, preventing complete reduction.

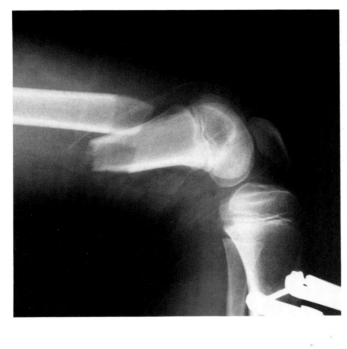
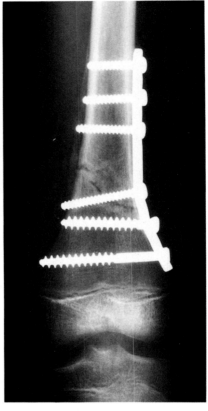

differentiate them from physeal separation (Fig. 25). Anatomically, the collateral ligaments and cruciate ligaments insert into the distal femoral epiphysis, leaving the distal femoral physis rather unprotected. Bending stress through the knee causes failure at the weakest link in the system. Given the same trauma, the young child tends to have a metaphyseal fracture, the adolescent a physeal injury, and the late teen a ligament injury. The tibial epiphysis is less likely to be injured because of the prolonged insertion of the collateral ligaments. Contrary to the assumption that all ligamentous insertion occurred on the tibial metaphysis, Ogden[74] has shown that there is a significant insertion of the ligamentous structure of the knee onto the tibial epiphysis. The patella tendon inserts into the anterior extension of the proximal tibia epiphysis, which can lead to avulsion of the tibial tubercle. The insertions of the cruciate ligaments into the anterior and posterior tibial spines predispose to avulsion injuries in these areas. In general, the tibial spine insertions are weaker than the femoral insertions of the cruciate ligaments or the ligaments themselves. Distal femoral epiphyseal fractures greatly outnumber proximal tibial epiphyseal inju-

FIGURE 25
Stress radiographs of the knee will differentiate between physeal fractures and rare ligamentous injury. **Left**, At rest and (**right**) with valgus stress showing medial instability.

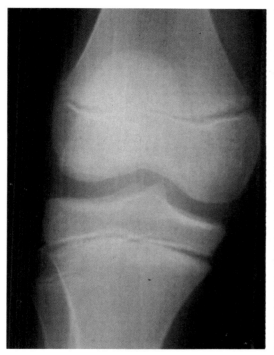
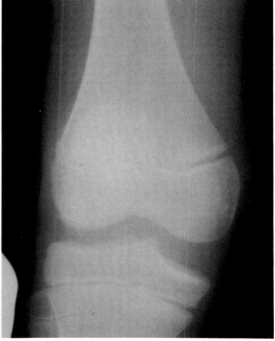

ries.[75,76] Meniscal injuries in the child's knee are relatively rare.[77]

In caring for knee injuries in children the general goals are: (1) Anatomic reduction of growth plates in those patients with significant growth remaining; (2) Anatomic reduction of articular surfaces (no vertical stepoff and less than 2 mm gap); and (3) Preservation of ligamentous attachments at anatomic length. In all cases with vascular compromise, the use of internal fixation is preferred, if possible, to provide a stable environment that will facilitate vascular repair.

DISTAL FEMORAL PHYSEAL FRACTURES

The Salter-Harris classification is the standard classification used to describe physeal and epiphyseal injuries.[78] The type I fracture is a transverse fracture through the growth plate with propagation into neither the epiphysis nor the metaphysis. Experimentally, such fractures tend to wander into the metaphysis and epiphysis rather than remain isolated to the physeal cartilage. The nondisplaced Salter I fracture is usually diagnosed by pain and tenderness over the physeal plate, with evidence of displacement on a stress view. In general, these are stable fractures that heal rapidly with a period of immobilization of three to four weeks. The risk of growth arrest in such an injury is minimal.

Displaced Salter I fractures require reduction and, at times, cross-pinning to obtain stability. If the fracture is stable, simple cast immobilization after reduction is all that is

FIGURE 26
This baby had a birth injury diagnosed as a physeal separation of the distal femur. Reduction and splinting are indicated in the acute injury. Growth arrest is rare, and remodeling is rapid.

FIGURE 27
The anteriorly displaced distal femoral epiphysis is usually unstable after reduction. Vascular injury can occur. Crossed pinning is the treatment of choice for fracture stabilization.

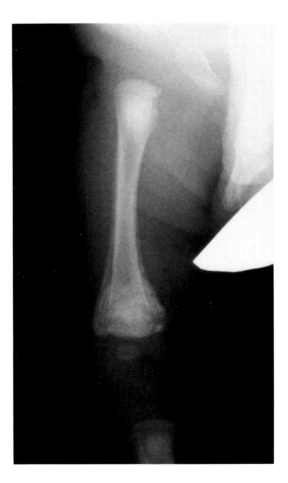

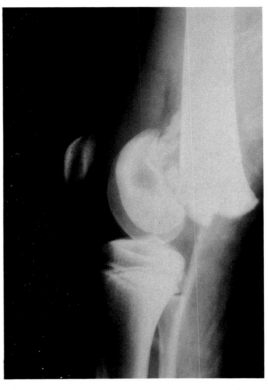

necessary. A "classic" Salter I distal femoral fracture occurs in a newborn as an obstetric fracture. After reduction, these fractures are generally stable and require only splinting. Growth arrest is rare, and remodeling is rapid (Fig. 26).

In the older child, the displaced distal femoral physeal fracture with medial, lateral, or posterior initial displacement is often stable following reduction. With anterior displacement of the Salter I fracture, instability is fre-

quently a problem (Fig. 27). To ensure stability, flexion of the knee to beyond 90 degrees is required, which is an unacceptable position of immobilization. Vascular injury may accompany this fracture, which makes cast immobilization less desirable. If cast immobilization is chosen, the fracture should be followed at three- to four-day intervals for two weeks to be sure that displacement has not occurred. An excellent and preferable method of stabilization is crossed K-wire pinning.

The technique for cross-pinning of the distal femoral epiphysis is shown in Figure 27. After reduction is obtained under fluoroscopic imaging, a small incision is made medially and laterally just posterior to the midline of the condyle. The AO tissue protector with jagged edge is placed at the margin of the articular surface and the medial or lateral bony epiphysis. The tissue protector, as the name implies, protects the soft tissue and also prevents the K-wire from sliding at the time of insertion. Wire insertion should be done under fluoroscopic control. The pin entry point should be just posterior to midcondyle, with the pins directed anteriorly at an angle of 10 to 15 degrees (Fig. 28). The pin should cross proximal to the physis, because crossing at the physis can lead to rotational instability. The pin is driven through the metaphysis to engage the opposite cortex and the end of the pin is bent and buried under the skin, because leaving the pins protruding through the skin can predispose to septic arthritis of the knee. Although the K-wires provide provisional internal fixation of these fractures, they must be supplemented with a cast. After a four-week period of immobilization, the patient can be started on a range-of-motion program. The pins can be removed shortly thereafter.

Salter II distal femoral fractures are frequent injuries in adolescents.[75,76] Growth arrest is relatively common secondary to a central area of physeal crush adjacent to the metaphyseal fragment (Fig. 29). The medial lateral and posterior fracture rarely is accompanied by vascular injury. However, the anterior displaced fracture is at high risk for injury to the popliteal artery and nerve. The peroneal nerve can also be injured, just as with the Salter I fracture. The anterior displaced Salter II is problematic and unstable unless placed in flexion approaching 90 degrees. Cross-pinning is the standard treatment for this fracture, as it is with the Salter I. In the young child, when a Salter II fracture is displaced medially, laterally, or posteriorly, closed reduction is often stable. In the young, thin child with good periosteum, a stable reduction may be satisfactorily held in a long leg cast. In more difficult cases, a spica may be required to fully immobilize this fracture.

An alternative treatment for unstable Salter II fractures with a large metaphyseal fragment (Thurston-Holland sign), is metaphyseal lag screw fixation. A lag screw is placed through the fragment and into the metaphysis (Fig. 30), either percutaneously, after closed re-

FIGURE 28

The entry point for crossed pins in the distal femoral epiphysis is just posterior to the midpoint of the femoral condyle. Pins should be aimed slightly anteriorly in the sagittal plane and should engage the opposite cortex after crossing the growth plate. Pins should cross well above the growth plate. The ends of the pins should be buried as they may penetrate the joint.

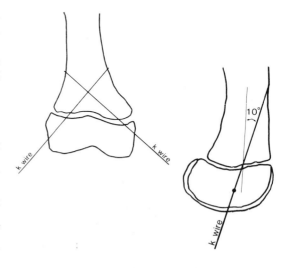

duction, or as an open procedure. A cannulated lag screw works best for this procedure, which is indicated only with large metaphyseal fragments. Lag screws should not be placed across the growth plate in children. This technique of fixation requires anatomic reduction under fluoroscopic control. A K-wire of appropriate size for a cannulated lag screw is then placed from the metaphyseal fragment into the proximal femoral metaphysis. Fixation is accomplished by placing the lag screw over the wire. In order to stabilize the fracture adequately, the threads of the screw must be fully in the proximal fragment—not crossing the fracture line. To use this technique of metaphyseal screw fixation, the metaphyseal fragment should be at least 2.5 cm long. Cast immobilization is always necessary, because the lag screw provides provisional stability and not rigid internal fixation. With a small metaphyseal fragment, if instability persists after closed reduction, closed K-wire fixation is used.

FIGURE 29

This Salter II fracture has a surprisingly high incidence of growth arrest, usually at the central area adjacent to the metaphyseal fragment. **Left**, Early central bone formation across the physis may be seen on plain radiograph tomography. **Right**, The growth plate has closed centrally six months postfracture.

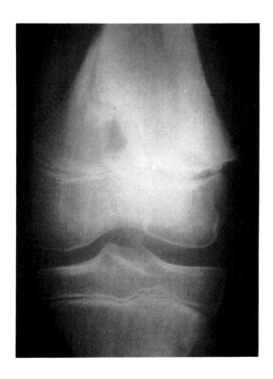
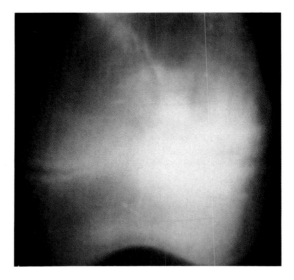

In the presence of multiple injuries or vascular compromise, internal fixation with either metaphyseal lag screws or crossed epiphyseal pinning is always indicated. Bony stability should be gained before attempting vascular repair. Because of the need for prompt revascularization of the extremity, bony fixation must be achieved rapidly. At present, too little is known to suggest that anatomic fixation of distal femoral physeal fractures will decrease the rate of growth arrest. This decrease has been shown convincingly in ankle fractures, however, and I suspect it is also true in the distal femur.

Distal femoral Salter III fractures (Fig. 31) are rare injuries, and they can be difficult to diagnose because the fracture is often minimally displaced. On an anteroposterior view, a vertical line is seen through the intracondylar notch. Occasionally, this can only be seen on a stress view of the knee of a patient with an acute hemarthrosis. The presence of fat in the knee aspirate suggests an intra-articular fracture, and a specific diagnosis of bony injury should certainly be pursued. A nondisplaced Salter III fracture on the anteroposterior view should be further evaluated with a computed tomography scan in all cases to allow proper visualization of the patellofemoral joint. The fracture displacement should be evaluated in terms of the width of the gap between the femoral condyles, as seen in the anteroposterior view, and also as an anterior open-book type of injury, where the patellofemoral joint may be significantly involved. A gap greater than 2 mm, or any vertical step off, is an indication for open reduction and internal fixation, because in this fracture anatomic alignment is critical.

FIGURE 30

A lag screw may be used (percutaneously) for stabilization if the metaphyseal fragment is large enough. Cast immobilization must supplement this fixation.

This acute Salter II fracture (**left**) is stabilized with lag screws through the metaphyseal fragment (**right**).

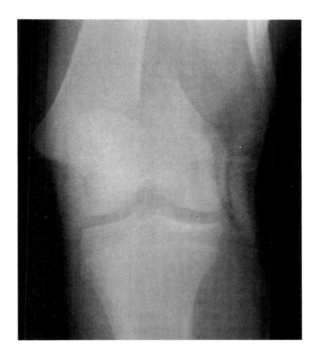
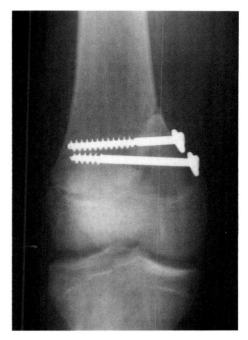

Open reduction and internal fixation of a Salter III distal femoral fracture (femoral condyle fracture) requires that the fracture be fixed anatomically, and that the blood supply to the femoral condyle be preserved. Because the fractured femoral condyle has a cleavage plane through the femoral notch, is bounded superiorly by a growth plate, and is almost entirely covered by articular cartilage, it is apparent that all blood supply to the condyle comes from its peripheral soft tissue. The area of blood supply is the relatively small space where the collateral ligament inserts and periosteum covers the medial and lateral aspect of the femoral condyle. Stripping of this soft tissue and periosteum to gain better exposure should be avoided because it will lead to osteonecrosis of the femoral condyle. There is room for one and maybe two screws lagging the displaced femoral condyle onto the intact opposite condyle. Screws should be placed to avoid violating the femoral notch. The screw should rest within the contralateral epiphysis and not encroach on the growth plate or the joint. Cast immobilization is required after fixation. One lag screw is generally sufficient to fix this fracture. In a case where both condyles are fractured, they should be lagged together, once the articular surface has been restored, and then secured to the shaft of the femur using crossed K-wires or plate fixation, depending on the growth remaining in the individual patient. Priorities in a severely comminuted or open fracture are, first, to try to reconstruct the articular surface and, second, to try to reconstruct the growth plate. Finally, the fractured fragment is attached to the shaft. Combinations of internal and external skeletal fixation are warranted in some severe cases.

A Salter IV fracture should be fixed, if it is unstable and/or displaced. Both the growth plate and the articular surface must be re-

FIGURE 31

Left, The Salter III fracture of the distal femoral epiphysis is occasionally obvious, as in this case, but at times shows only as a small vertical line, visible only on stress views. **Right**, Demonstrates reduction with lag screws to the stable femoral condyle.

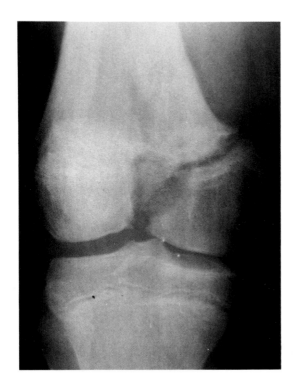
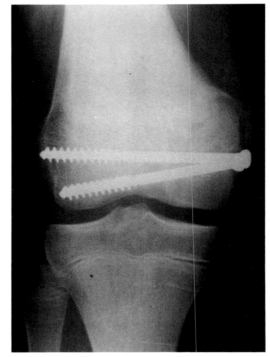

duced anatomically. Nothing less than perfect reduction is acceptable in this fracture. The preferred method of fixation is with transverse lag screws through the metaphyseal fragment and the epiphyseal fragment. The technique previously described for the use of lag screws in the metaphysis and epiphysis is used. For some comminuted displaced fractures, it is necessary to prioritize treatment goals as stated above (Fig. 32).

All distal femoral epiphyseal fractures heal rapidly in three to four weeks. Stiffness is a problem with prolonged immobilization, and immobilization should not exceed four weeks. All of these fractures should be followed for the possibility of growth arrest. Growth arrest is a major long-term complication of physeal fractures. All injuries to the growth plate should be followed for growth abnormality. Adolescents have a high rate of growth arrest even after diaphyseal fractures in the lower extremity.

AVULSION FRACTURES ABOUT THE KNEE

Avulsion fractures about the knee may involve the collateral or cruciate ligaments and the patellar tendon. These fractures are more common than injuries to the ligaments themselves. Just as ligament injuries to the knee in adults are often associated with diaphyseal fractures, avulsion injuries can occur with femoral and tibial fractures in children.[67] A radiograph of the knee joint should be carefully evaluated in all diaphyseal fractures of the lower extremity.

FIGURE 32

In a severely comminuted distal femoral fracture, reduce the articular surfaces first, then the growth plate. Finally, deal with the supracondylar component of the fracture. Obtaining a stable articular surface takes precedence over physeal preservation, as in this case, where a plate spans the physis. The plate will be removed as soon as possible. In severe injuries, it is necessary to prioritize treatment goals.

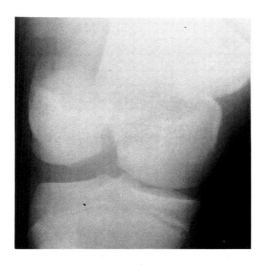

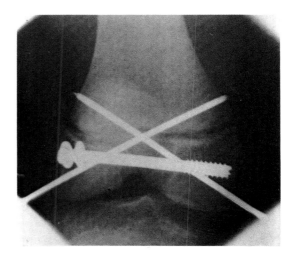

THE TIBIAL SPINE FRACTURE

The anterotibial spine fracture is the most common fracture of this type. The insertion of the anterior cruciate ligament (ACL) into the anterotibial spine is much broader than a simple insertion onto the bony tibial spine itself. The mechanism of injury resembles an ACL rupture in an adult, and the tibial spine with adjacent articular cartilage is displaced. A stretch injury to the ACL substance may accompany this injury, but ACL rupture is not reported in association with tibial spine injury. As shown in Figure 33, this fracture is classified as type I, II, or III, based on degree of displacement of the fragment.[79-81] Closed reduction is accomplished by extending the knee fully, which usually requires general anesthesia. This is usually accompanied by knee aspiration to relieve pain and facilitate placement in extension. The leg is then placed in a cylinder or a long leg case, and radiographs are taken to evaluate the position of the tibial spine (Fig. 34). Reduction is obtained as the femoral condyle rolls forward and pushes on the

FIGURE 33

The commonly used classification of tibial spine fracture: **(left)** type I, nondisplaced, **(center)** type II, hinged, and **(right)** type III, totally displaced. (Reproduced with permission from Rang M: Knee joint. *Children's Fractures,* ed 2. Philadelphia, JB Lippincott, 1982, p 288.)

articular component of the tibial spine fragment. Even though full extension increases the tension on the ACL and, therefore, can increase tension on the fracture fragment, the extension method of reduction is best. If the knee is immobilized in a flexed position, the articular extension of this fracture fragment will remain elevated and will cause

FIGURE 34
This displaced fracture (**left**) may be reduced by placing the knee in full extension in a cylinder cast (**right**).

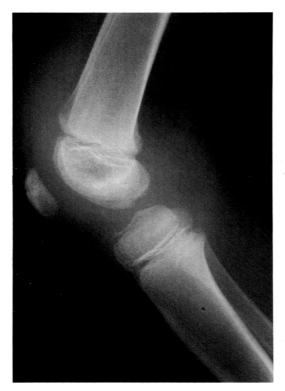
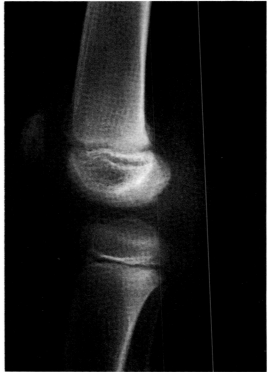

a flexion deformity of the knee when the fracture heals. The duration of immobilization for this fracture is four to six weeks.

Surgical treatment of a displaced tibial spine fracture is indicated for the type III injury that fails to reduce with extension of the knee. In many cases, this failure to reduce is seen best on lateral tomography after an extension cast is applied. The methods for achieving internal fixation at the time of open reduction[82] or arthroscopy vary. A skilled arthroscopist can obtain reduction and fixation of the fragment using a K-wire or a small screw. The K-wire is left subcutaneously and removed later, when the fracture has healed. Because of its position, the tibial spine is hard to fix with a K-wire in less than 90 degrees of flexion. Care must be taken to be sure that the K-wire will

not impinge on an articular surface when the knee is extended to 30 degrees of flexion for immobilization. For this reason, a small intraepiphyseal screw may be preferable to the K-wire (Fig. 35). Meniscal tear in association with this fracture is rare.

Open reduction of the tibial fragment is done through a small medial arthrotomy. The tibial spine fracture is reduced with direct pressure and may be fixed using either a suture technique, K-wire technique, or a small AO screw, which remains intraepiphyseal. Each technique has its advocates, and it is hard to recommend one over another. The AO screw should be short enough to remain intraepiphyseal. In the suture technique, the intraepiphyseal suture can be brought out through holes drilled underneath the patellar tendon.

FIGURE 35
Failing closed reduction, the type III tibial spine fracture may require open reduction and internal fixation with a suture, a screw, or a K-wire. In this case, a suture was used.

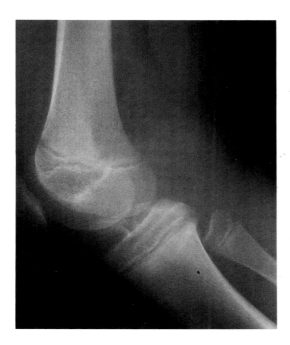
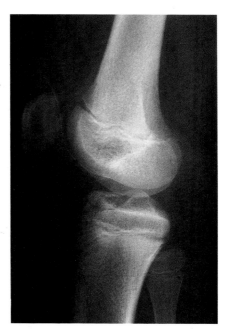

A nonresorbable suture or wires are generally used for this, however, the fracture will heal rapidly and a strong resorbable suture (not catgut) can be used without problems. Postoperative immobilization is four weeks. Despite anatomic fixation of a tibial spine fracture, laxity of the knee joint may exist after surgery. This may be secondary to a stretch injury to the ligament in association with bony avulsion. I have not seen symptomatic instability after anatomic fixation of this tibial spine fragment.

AVULSION OF THE POSTERIOR CRUCIATE LIGAMENT (PCL)

PCL avulsion occurs rarely, but it should be recognized and repaired promptly when it does.[79,83,84] Patients with this injury have an acutely swollen knee that is held in 30 to 40 degrees of flexion. Radiographs generally show a bony avulsion off the posterior aspect of the tibial epiphysis (Fig. 36). The anteroposterior radiograph shows the fragment to be in the midst of the femoral notch. A lateral radiograph can help to identify this, but a computed tomography scan is most accurate.

Late presentation of PCL avulsions with instability have not been seen or reported, but, because the injury is quite rare, it is suspected that they may exist without being recognized. Anatomic replacement of the bony fragment and PCL is indicated and is done through a posterior Henry approach to the knee. Once the fragment is identified and has been replaced provisionally, with K-wire fixation, an intraepiphyseal screw is used to fix the fragment (Fig. 36). Because the central posterior location of this fragment is adjacent to the neu-

FIGURE 36

The PCL avulsion should be repaired open using an intraepiphyseal screw for fixation. **Top left,** The avulsed fragment is best seen on the lateral view (*arrows*) but may be best demonstrated on computed tomography (**bottom**). If displaced, open reduction with internal fixation is indicated (**top right**).

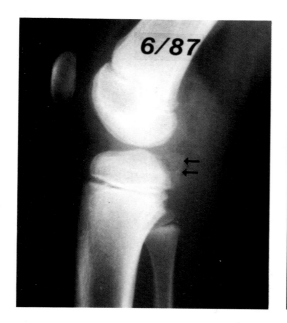
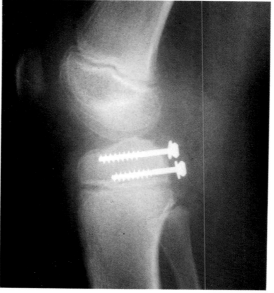
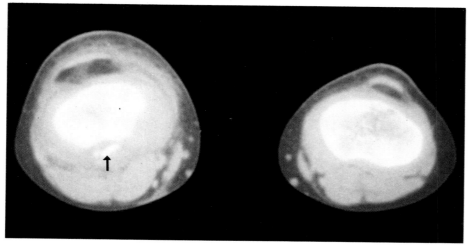

rovascular bundle, arthroscopic replacement or percutaneous pinning of the fragment is contraindicated. The patient should be immobilized in a cast or splint for about four weeks. Early motion can be begun if stable fixation is obtained, but, in general, immobilization is well tolerated in this patient population.

AVULSION OF COLLATERAL LIGAMENTS AND CAPSULE

Avulsion of the insertion of the posterolateral capsule and collateral ligament has been described by Brunner[85] and others (Fig. 37). It can occur either as a primary injury or in association with displaced femoral or tibial diaphyseal fracture. The fracture, which is hard to visualize on plain radiographs, is best seen on an oblique film. The fragment is at the posterolateral corner of the distal femoral epiphysis. If the fracture fragment is displaced, there is a high risk of growth arrest (Fig. 37). Anatomic reduction of this fragment or excision of a smaller fragment is indicated to prevent growth arrest. If a collateral ligament is avulsed with attached bony fragment, replacement with a percutaneous or an open fixation technique is indicated.

TIBIAL TUBERCLE AVULSION

Tibial tubercle avulsion (Fig. 38) is an injury of the adolescent knee joint that occurs just before the end of growth. This fracture usually occurs with jumping, either at push off or at landing. It is usually an isolated injury. It has been classified as types I, II, and III (Fig. 39).[86,87] The type I injury can be treated with a cast only. Types II and III injuries require surgical treatment. The type II lesion maintains an intact superior contact between the avulsed portion of the tibial tubercle and the remaining portion of the tibial epiphysis. The articular surface of the knee remains intact and meniscal injury is very rare. In a type III injury, the tibial tubercle is avulsed with fracture through the articular surface and, at times, disruption of the menisci. Surgical treatment of the type II lesion requires reduction of the fragment and pinning without need for exploration of the knee joint. Internal fixation is best accomplished with one or two screws through the tibial tubercle into the proximal tibia. Because this fracture generally occurs just at the end of growth, the risk of significant growth arrest is nil. If significant growth does remain, fixation with a smooth K-wire technique will allow growth to continue and will prevent recurvatum. An alternative approach, which depends on the growth remaining, is screw fix-

FIGURE 37
Watch for the avulsion fracture at the posterolateral corner of the distal femoral epiphysis (arrows). This fracture can occur in association with a diaphyseal fracture. Growth arrest is a common sequela of this injury.

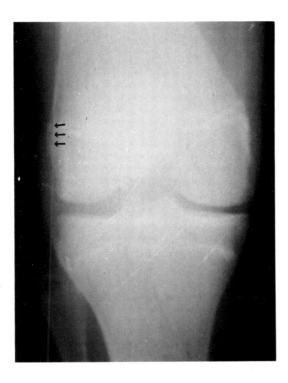

ation of the tibial tubercle and proximal tibial epiphysiodesis. The approach for screw fixation is a direct anterior approach that splits the patellar tendon for access to the tibial tubercle fragment but keeps dissection of the tendon insertion to a minimum. Anatomic reduction of the fracture should be confirmed on radiograph. Care should be taken that the screw is, if anything, inclined proximally and posteriorly. The screw should not be aimed distally, because it might tend to pull out.

In the type III fracture, the joint is disrupted and there is a possibility of comminution of the articular surface as well as meniscal abnormalities (Fig. 40). Therefore, joint arthrotomy and joint exploration is indicated at the time of open reduction of the tibial tubercle

FIGURE 38
The tibial tubercle avulsion is an injury of
the nearly mature skeleton. It is frequently
associated with jumping.

FIGURE 39
The classification of tibial spine fractures is
as follows: **Left**, Type I, minimal
displacement; **Center**, Type II, hinged
displacement without joint involvement; and
Right, Type III, displacement with joint
involvement.

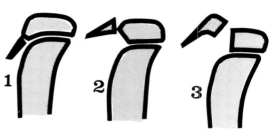

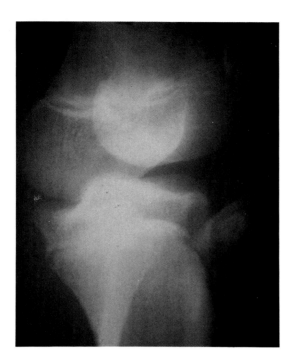

fragment. The best surgical approach is
through an anteromedial incision with a small
medial parapatellar arthrotomy to visualize the
joint surface. The distal portion of the patellar
tendon can be split longitudinally for screw
placement. The insertion of the patellar tendon should be maintained on the tibial tubercle fragment. After the fracture is identified
and reduced with provisional K-wire fixation,
radiographs should be taken to ensure that anatomic reduction of the joint surface has been
obtained. Any small comminuted fragments of
the articular surface should be held in place
with K-wires or small screws at the time of
fixation. If the menisci obscure the evaluation
of the joint surface, as is often the case, an
approach to visualize the articular surface is
under the meniscus by transecting the anterior
portion of the meniscotibial ligament. This exposure facilitates observation of the joint surface as the meniscus is retracted superiorly.
Meniscal tears can be repaired and articular
surface continuity ensured. The meniscotibial
ligament should be repaired after this approach and the tibial tubercle solidly fixed in
place.

The position of screws and bone fragments
should be confirmed on radiograph. The fracture should be immobilized for three to four
weeks and physical therapy begun. In the
management of a comminuted intra-articular
fracture, continuous passive motion may be of
value in the healing of the joint surface if stable internal fixation is obtained.

PROXIMAL TIBIAL PHYSEAL INJURIES

Proximal tibial physeal injuries are relatively rare, because the collateral ligaments
and capsule have a broad metaphyseal insertion onto the tibia.[88-92] The lateral collateral
ligament inserts into the proximal fibula.
There is a capsular insertion, as pointed out
by Ogden,[74] onto the tibial epiphysis, which
does predispose to epiphyseal fracturing, but
the incidence is low. The goal of treatment for
displaced epiphyseal fracture of the proximal
tibia is similar to that in the distal femur in
that anatomic reduction of the articular surface
and growth plate should be achieved. If the
distal metaphyseal segment in a Salter I or II

FIGURE 40
The proximal tibial physis is rarely injured, but, with displacement of the metaphysis posteriorly, there is a high probability of vascular injury. Rapid reduction, stabilization, and vascular evaluation are indicated. K-wires provide the best form of fixation.

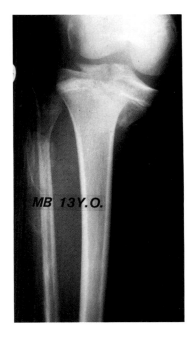 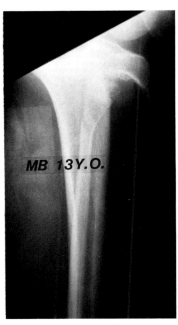 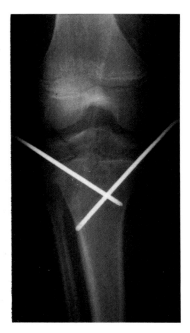

fracture is displaced posteriorly, there is a high risk of injuries to the popliteal vessel and peroneal nerve. The soft-tissue injury and risk of compartment syndrome is of utmost importance in displaced proximal tibial fractures. Stabilization, using crossed K-wires, should be obtained as rapidly as possible to facilitate management of the soft-tissue problem.

Salter IV fractures and tibial plateau fractures occur in teenagers. Reduction of the articular surface and stabilization with interfragmentary screw fixation or a buttress plate is necessary. The first goal is to achieve an intact articular surface, the second is to restore the growth plate to maintain alignment.

OSTEOCHONDRAL FRACTURES

Osteochondral fractures occur in adolescents either secondary to external trauma directly over the femoral condyle or by pressure of the patella on the femoral condyle in the process of dislocation.[93-95] The osteochondral fracture may involve either the femoral condyle or the patella. Tibial osteochondral fractures are associated with cruciate ligament avulsion or type III tibial tubercle avulsion, as previously discussed.

An osteochondral fracture should be suspected in an adolescent with an acute hemarthrosis. The finding of fat in a knee aspirate further supports the diagnosis of fracture. Plain radiograph reveals a thin line of bone (Fig. 41) corresponding to the tangential view of the cortical component of the osteochondral fragment. Viewed enface, the fragment is generally so small that minimal roentgenographic image is apparent. A computed tomography scan and magnetic resonance imaging may help define the extent of the lesion. Misdiagnosis will result in loose body and loss

FIGURE 41
Osteochondral fractures are seen on plain radiograph as a "wisp" of bone (arrows). These fractures frequently can be seen only when viewed tangentially.

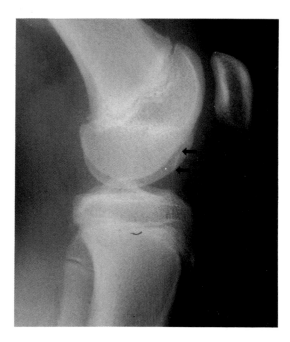

of the opportunity to reconstruct the articular surface.

Once diagnosed, the treatment is repair of the defect, either arthroscopically or surgically, or excision of the fragment. If the fragment is on a weightbearing surface and has any attached bone, it should be repaired. If an osteochondral fragment involves a nonweightbearing portion of articular cartilage, excision of the fragment is probably preferable. Fixation of the fragment should be with steel pins or resorbable pins. There is not sufficient experience with resorbable pins at this time to recommend them, although some are being used. Herbert screws have also been used for repair of osteochondral fragments. Generally, because the fragments are small and poorly secured despite internal fixation, immobilization is mandatory. If the lesion is excised, the joint is not immobilized, and early motion should be begun. There is insufficient infor-

mation in the literature on osteochondral fractures on which to base a firm recommendation for fixation technique and postoperative management, but common practice is to stabilize the lesion as described, followed by immobilization and physical therapy.

PATELLA FRACTURES

Patella fractures occur either because of direct trauma over the patella or as an avulsion injury of the inferior, superior, or lateral margin. As was mentioned previously, an osteochondral fracture of the articular surface of the patella may occur during dislocation. Comminution of the patella, a frequent consequence of trauma in adults, is relatively rare in children. Bipartite patellas[96-98] occur, with a secondary ossification center in the superior lateral corner of the patella. With a fracture through the synchondrosis, this can become symptomatic, but this injury is rarely displaced. The symptomatic bipartite patella, presumably posttraumatic, may be treated by restriction of activity or brief immobilization for symptomatic treatment.

The displaced patella fractures are usually transverse, with associated disruption of the quadriceps mechanism. In transverse patella fractures, with displacement of less than 2 mm and no vertical stepoff in the articular cartilage, treatment is simple cast immobilization in a long leg cylinder. If the fractured patella is displaced more than 2 mm, open reduction with internal fixation is indicated. Tension banding (Fig. 42) or cerclage wiring remains the treatment of choice for this fracture.

The patella "sleeve fracture" is an unusual injury that is seen only in children.[99] It is an avulsion injury of the inferior pole of the patella with a variable amount of articular cartilage attached. The injury occurs with sudden giving way of the knee, usually associated with a hemarthrosis. There is a palpable gap at the inferior pole of the patella and a high-riding patella with absent knee extension. The avulsed fracture fragment has minimal bone and is often difficult to see on radiographs. It may be separated completely from the patella. A high-riding patella is highly suggestive of this injury.

If the "sleeve fracture" is nondisplaced, simple immobilization is the only treatment required. If it is displaced with quadriceps disruption, open reduction with internal fixation is indicated as recommended by Houghton and Ackroyd.[99] Although osteonecrosis of the patella and fragmentation of the articular cartilage have been reported with this injury following open reduction, it is nonetheless clear that surgical repair of the displaced sleeve fracture is required.

SUMMARY

In summary, fractures about the knee include the growth-plate injuries with accompanying metaphyseal and epiphyseal fractures, avulsion fracture, osteochondral fractures, and patella fractures. The approach to these injuries requires anatomic reduction of articular surfaces, reattachment of avulsed tendons by open or closed means, and anatomic and nearly anatomic restoration of physeal injuries. In the child and adolescent, rehabilitation to regain motion and strength after a significant knee injury generally involves physical therapy. Ideally, the period of immobilization will not exceed four weeks.

TIBIA FRACTURES IN CHILDREN

Although the tibia is one of the most frequently fractured bones in the child, certain anatomic regions are rarely injured and present special challenges when they are. In addition, infants and young children display healing properties different from those of adolescents (who can often be treated as adults, depending on amount of growth remaining), and treatment programs must be adjusted appropriately. This discussion of tibia fractures will deal with three anatomic areas—the proximal tibial epiphysis (excluding tibial tubercle avulsions), the proximal metaphysis, and the tibial shaft. Injuries that may require surgical intervention will be highlighted.

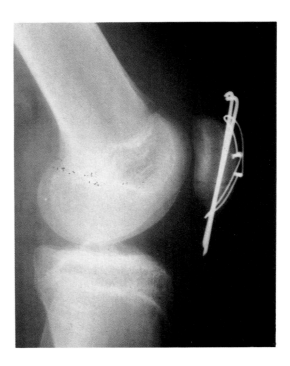

FIGURE 42
Technique of tension banding of the patella as used in adults is appropriate for children when open reduction is required.

PROXIMAL TIBIAL EPIPHYSIS

Anatomy and Pathology

Fractures of the tibia through the proximal epiphyseal cartilage are rare, accounting for fewer than 1% of all epiphyseal injuries, despite the frequent exposure of the child's knee to trauma. Stability of the proximal epiphysis is largely conferred by the irregular shape of the physis, with an anterior-downward extension of the tibial tuberosity, and by the many musculotendinous units that cross the knee without inserting on the epiphysis (gastrocnemius, biceps femoris, and medial hamstrings). In addition, the lateral collateral ligament largely inserts on the fibula rather than on the tibial epiphysis, and the medial collateral ligament inserts on both the epiphysis and metaphysis, which provides further stability for this region. Because the popliteal artery exits the popliteal space in close proximity to

FIGURE 43
The distal tibial segment is displaced posteriorly in this type I proximal epiphyseal fracture. Vascular occlusion is possible. (Redrawn with permission from Mayo Foundation.)

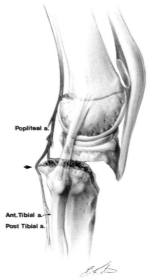

Popliteal a.

Ant. Tibial a.
Post Tibial a.

the proximal tibial epiphysis, displaced fractures in this region can produce both acute and delayed vascular injury (Fig. 43).

The mechanism of injury is usually a direct force applied to the knee, as can occur in a motor vehicle accident or in sports related activities where the knee is forcibly hyperextended or abducted. This injury is to be distinguished from tibial tubercle avulsions, which are largely caused by indirect forces generated by sudden muscular contractions about the knee. The peak age distribution is at 14 years of age, notably close to the time of physeal closure. Burkhart and Peterson[90] have also identified a younger group of children (aged 2–6 years) that sustained direct injury to the proximal tibial epiphysis from lawn mower accidents.

The clinical evaluation should include a detailed neurovascular examination with rapid institution of treatment if vascular compromise exists. Vascular status also must be monitored at regular intervals so that late arterial thrombosis can be identified. If apparent knee instability is present during clinical examination, stress radiographs will be necessary to distinguish ligamentous injury from physeal separation.

Classification and Treatment

All types of growth-plate injuries can be seen in the proximal tibia, and the Salter-Harris system sufficiently illustrates them (Fig. 44). Most injuries to this region are type II physeal separations, and when displacement occurs it is usually in a posterolateral or posteromedial direction. Type I injuries are the second most common pattern of injury and may be difficult to identify if nondisplaced. When displacement occurs, the distal fragment moves posteriorly toward the neurovascular bundle (Fig. 45).

Closed reduction should be performed for all type I and type II fractures, after which the stability is assessed. These fractures are frequently unstable and require some form of internal fixation, which can consist of crossed smooth Steinman pins. In type II separations in which the metaphyseal fragment (Thurston-Holland sign) is large enough, a cancellous screw can be placed across the metaphysis, which avoids crossing the physis with wires. In the adolescent, insufficient growth remains to correct any residual deformity following an imprecise reduction, and fractures treated without surgery must be watched closely for late displacement. Pins are left in place for 4 to 6 weeks, and the knee should be immobilized during this period.

Displaced type III injuries require precise internal fixation, and this is accomplished with a horizontal transphyseal lag screw. Usually, two parallel 4.0-mm cancellous screws are used. Generally, type IV fractures should be treated in a similar fashion, even if the fragments are minimally displaced, in order to prevent later development of joint surface incongruity and subsequent physeal bar formation.

The presence of a vascular injury is an absolute indication for internal fixation to avoid subsequent damage to the arterial repair that could occur during further manipulation of the leg. This treatment plan is also instituted if arteriography is planned after fracture manipulation to ensure that the reduction is not lost. Reconstitution of arterial flow can result

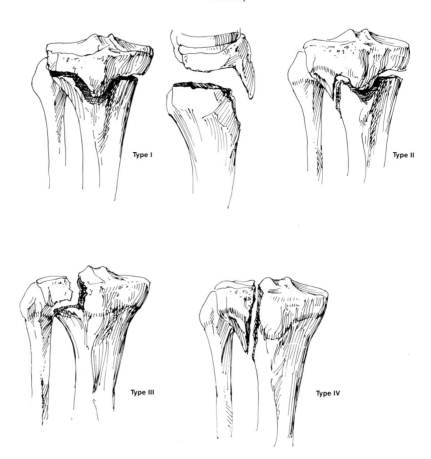

FIGURE 44
Salter-Harris classification for proximal tibial epiphyseal fractures. In types II, III, and IV fracture patterns, the displaced fragment may be lateral, as illustrated, or located medially.

in a reperfusion compartment syndrome. This condition is best treated by prophylactic complete fasciotomy, and it must be carefully monitored.

Complications

Fortunately, because many of these injuries occur during adolescence, the risk of significant growth deformities is small. However, it should be noted that there is a much higher incidence of growth disturbance with type I and type II fracture patterns than is normally expected with this fracture pattern. This prob-

lem is more likely to occur if a hyperextension force was responsible for the fracture displacement, presumably due to shearing across the physeal layer. Shelton and Canale[91] reported a 25% incidence of 1 cm or more growth retardation in those patients with types I and II epiphyseal fractures. In their series, no significant growth deformity occurred with type III and type IV patterns, most of which were surgically restored to anatomic realignment and stabilized.

However, premature growth arrest in a type III or IV pattern can result in a varus or valgus

FIGURE 45
A type I epiphyseal fracture; radiographs
of injury (**left**) and after pinning (**right**).

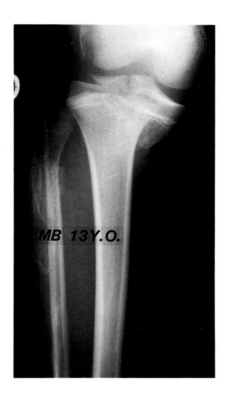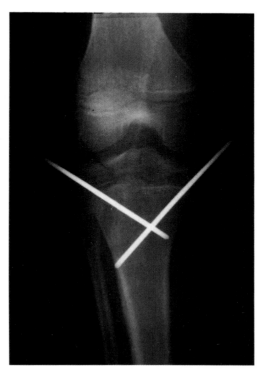

deformity, as well as recurvatum. Burkhart and Peterson[90] reported growth disturbance in 9 of 27 patients (33%), the majority of whom had type IV fractures. Two children eventually required amputation; in one case because of unrecognized compartment syndrome, and in the other as a result of prolonged vascular insufficiency. These two cases are examples of the potential for catastrophic complications with this type of fracture.

PROXIMAL TIBIAL METAPHYSIS

Metaphyseal fractures of the proximal tibia are fairly common injuries in the 2- to 8-year-old age group and are generally not difficult to treat. Motor vehicle accidents are the usual mechanism for injury in displaced fractures, and fibular fracture may also be present. Pro-nounced initial displacement is uncommon, and subsequent healing is usually rapid and complete with closed management. However, despite their often relatively innocuous appearance, these fractures can be followed by a significant progressive valgus deformity of the leg. This deformity can even occur in minimally displaced fractures that have been carefully followed, and there is no way to predict whether or not this problem will develop. The severity of valgus angulation peaks at four to six months after injury and the angulation seems to stabilize after one year. The exact etiology remains somewhat obscure, and many theories have been offered,[100-102] although the most likely explanation is a selective overgrowth of the medial tibia secondary to asymmetric vascular stimulation.[100,101] Torus fractures of the proximal metaphysis are not known to produce this deformity.

Treatment should be directed toward a complete reduction with elimination of the medial gap and valgus angulation. If a medial space persists, open reduction is indicated, in order to remove any interposed periosteum or other soft tissues, with the hope that valgus angulation will not develop. Unfortunately, because there is no guarantee that the leg will remain straight, the family should be apprised of the potential for growth problems. Although many authors state that angulation of more than 15 degrees is an indication for corrective osteotomy,[103] this procedure carries a high risk of such perioperative problems as compartment syndrome, as well as recurrence of the deformity. Other authors have suggested that adequate remodeling can occur, especially through the distal tibial physis, and they advise delaying any surgical correction until the child is closer to maturity.[102,104]

It is important to note that proximal metaphyseal fractures are at high risk for development of elevated compartment pressures. This is especially true in the adolescent and in cases in which high-energy impact was the mechanism of injury. Figure 46 illustrates a proximal metaphyseal tibia fracture that was treated with external fixation after the extremity underwent complete fasciotomy for an associated compartment syndrome.

FRACTURE OF THE TIBIAL SHAFT

Anatomy and Pathology

Tibial diaphyseal fractures are the most common injury of the lower extremity in children. The type of fracture depends largely on the age of the child and the mechanism of injury. In infants and young children, because the tibial shaft is more porous, it is more likely to bend or buckle than it is to comminute. In addition, the surrounding periosteum is very thick, which imparts stability to the fracture and limits displacement. Also, most fractures are caused by indirect trauma (torsion), and the fibula is frequently intact. In older children and adolescents, the tibial shaft has its typical triangular shape in cross section, and it is composed of dense cortical bone with a somewhat less tenacious periosteum. This more mature anatomy is associated with different fracture patterns, and comminution and fragment displacement are more common. As can be expected, healing rates are correspondingly different, taking up to three to four months, as opposed to the average ten weeks in uncomplicated cases. Children with closed head injury also have delayed healing, averaging 12 to 14 weeks in closed fractures and 20 weeks in open injuries.[105]

The popliteal artery passes from the popliteal fossa between the two heads of the gastrocnemius and trifurcates just below the level of the fibular physeal plate. The anterotibial artery passes through the interosseous membrane and courses distally, closely applied to the membrane. The four anterior muscles of the leg lie in a fascial compartment between this anterior intermuscular septum and the tibia and are also bordered by the fibula. The deep peroneal nerve courses through this compartment with the artery. This anatomy is significant, because it relates to the development of the anterior compartment syndrome. The lateral compartment of the leg consists of the peroneal muscles; the posterior compartment contains the gastrocnemius-soleus group, posterior tibialis, and long toe flexors. The posterotibial artery and nerve are isolated from the tibial shaft and are protected from damage by the surrounding muscles. Hence, direct vascular disruption in tibia fractures is a rare occurrence in children, but neurovascular status must be routinely and carefully assessed.

Direct trauma to the tibia produces transverse fracture patterns with varying degrees of comminution, depending on the amount of force involved. Motor vehicle accidents are the most common cause of these high-energy fractures. Frequently the fibula is fractured, too, which makes the leg less stable. In the adolescent, sports-related injuries are the next most common mechanism for tibial shaft fractures, followed by falls from a height. The subcutaneous position of the tibial shaft makes it particularly susceptible to injury from direct forces.

Classification and Closed Management

There is no specific classification system that is particularly helpful in the treatment of tibial

FIGURE 46
Left, Despite the minimal displacement of this proximal metaphyseal fracture, a compartment syndrome developed. **Right**, External fixation was used after fasciotomy, allowing for subsequent wound care without compromising fracture alignment.

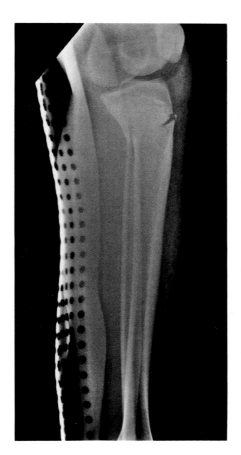
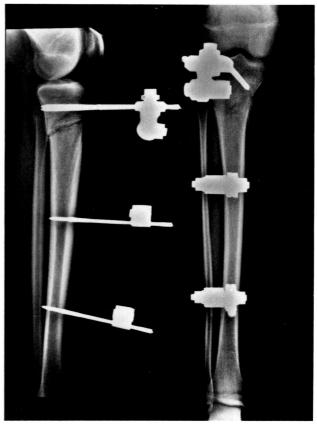

fractures; rather, it is of more benefit to describe the anatomic location, the fracture pattern, the amount of displacement and shortening, and the magnitude of soft-tissue injury. In addition, the mechanism of injury and the presence of an associated fibular fracture help to characterize the severity of the trauma. Mild injuries generally have less than 50% diaphyseal offset, minimal angulation, and no soft-tissue damage. Moderate injuries may have greater fracture displacement with angulation and grade I open soft-tissue wounds. Severe fractures usually show comminution, marked displacement, and grade II to III soft-tissue

damage. More severe injuries take longer to heal and have a higher incidence of complications.

Early assessment of the stability of the fracture pattern is also necessary, and some generalizations can be offered. Simply stated, unstable fractures tend to shorten, and in most cases the fibula is also fractured. Comminution or segmental fracture may be present (possibly with bone loss), the soft tissues are disrupted, and the mechanism of injury involves violent forces. Conversely, an intact fibula often confers stability to the tibia and although angulation may be difficult to control, significant shortening usually is not seen. Low energy fractures, especially in children younger than 6 years of age, are typically stable. Transverse, short oblique, and midshaft spiral fracture patterns are characteristic, and closed reduction with improved bone contact imparts more stability. An exception to this description of a stable fracture is the spiral fracture of the distal tibial diaphysis. In this case, if initial displacement of greater than one half of the shaft width has occurred, the primary reduction position is rarely retained, probably as a result of disruption of the interosseous membrane. In addition, dorsiflexion of the foot to a neutral position may produce an unacceptable recurvatum deformity. Surgical intervention may be necessary, especially in the adolescent.

Closed management of tibial shaft fractures in children, with casting, is the usual treatment and is appropriate for all stable fracture patterns. Ideally, the fracture is an isolated injury with no more than grade I open soft-tissue damage. Successful results are usually obtained, provided that the following features of tibial healing are well understood.

Growth Acceleration Periosteal stripping, followed by extensive callus formation and a subsequent increase in local blood supply, leads to an increase in the growth rate after childhood long-bone fractures. The ability to compensate for initial shortening decreases with age, with children younger than 5 years of age showing the greatest capacity and those older than 10 years displaying the least. However, unlike the fractured femur, this increase in tibial growth rate is less dramatic and predictable, and growth acceleration greater than 5 to 7 mm is unusual. In fact, in a review of 142 tibia fractures, Shannak[106] reported an average of only 4.35 mm of growth acceleration; thus, up to 10 mm shortening of the fractured leg can be tolerated if the goal is to get within 5 mm of the length of the other leg. Long spiral fractures and those with comminution will display more than average growth acceleration.

Open reduction and internal fixation of tibial fractures may result in overgrowth of the injured extremity, but this stimulatory effect generally does not last more than one year. The magnitude of tibial overgrowth with anatomic reduction and internal or external fixation is also greatest with comminuted or segmental injuries. Overgrowth is not routinely seen in girls aged 8 years or older, or in boys older than 10 years.

Remodeling Angular deformity can also correct spontaneously with growth; however, the final axial alignment should fall within 5 degrees varus or valgus. Obviously, infants and young children can remodel greater degrees of deformity, and in this age group approximately 50% of the angulation will correct. Although some remodeling occurs at the diaphysis through convex bone resorption, most angular compensation is achieved at the physeal level through asymmetrical longitudinal growth. Therefore, residual diaphyseal deformity may persist. In children older than 10 years, one can expect only about 25% of the axial malalignment to improve with subsequent growth. Shannak[106] demonstrated that one third of children with more than 10 degrees of angulation at healing had persistence of the malunion. Hansen and associates[107] reported only a 13.5% correction of angular deformity with subsequent growth.

Varus malalignment (up to 15 degrees in children) seems to remodel more completely than valgus deformity, but may be more poorly compensated for at the level of the foot and ankle. Recurvatum deformity also remodels poorly, and 10 degrees is the maximum that can be accepted at the time of initial healing. The combination of recurvatum with varus or valgus malunion should be prevented, because this condition has the least capacity to remodel to normal. Healing in malrotation is a permanent deformity.

INDICATIONS FOR SURGICAL TREATMENT

Most childhood tibial fractures can be managed satisfactorily by closed techniques; however, there are several clinical situations for which surgical stabilization is preferred. Such factors as the age of the patient, the severity of the fracture, other associated injuries, and expected healing rates must all be considered when designing a treatment plan.

Failure of Closed Management

During the course of closed treatment, if unacceptable position of the extremity persists, a poor result can be predicted based on the guidelines previously established for remodeling and growth acceleration capacity. Typically, this is most likely to occur in an adolescent with an unstable fracture pattern, where only minimal shortening (5–7 mm) and minor angulation (5 degrees) can be tolerated. External fixators provide a simple means of restoring alignment and length, with minimal soft-tissue disruption, and they can be replaced later by casting, as soon as early healing is evident on radiographs. Closed segmental fractures in which axial loading is not possible can also be difficult to control with casting alone, and external fixation may also be indicated in these cases.

Internal fixation with compression plates is rarely necessary. In a spiral or long oblique fracture pattern, fixation with lag screws, without plates, is possible and can be combined with casting or with external fixation.

Soft-Tissue Injury

Open fractures of the tibia, notably grade III severity, require external fixation in order to facilitate wound management. Soft-tissue defects combined with unstable fracture patterns (e.g., bone loss or segmental fracture), which are prone to shortening, are especially appropriate for external fixation (Fig. 47). Prolonged healing rates are to be expected, averaging 4 to 5 months, and the incidence of infection is similar to reported adult rates.[26] Early autologous bone grafting is recommended for bone defects once soft-tissue healing is complete.

Major vascular disruption occurs in 5% of open tibial fractures, and this situation is an absolute indication for surgical fracture intervention in order to protect the vascular repair and to stabilize the surrounding soft tissues. Either internal or external fixation can be used, depending on the extent of associated soft-tissue damage and the amount of time needed to apply the implant. Obviously, time is of the essence, and the surgeon should choose the technique that is most familiar.

Children with extensive burns of the lower extremity, associated with long bone fractures, are also candidates for external fixation. These devices obviously facilitate burn dressings and wound management, and they can be extended across adjacent joints to prevent contracture formation (Fig. 48).

Compartment Syndrome

Compartment syndrome occurs most often after what appears to be a relatively minor tibial fracture. The interosseous membrane remains intact, which allows for a rapid increase in anterior compartment tissue pressure caused by hemorrhage and edema. The typical fracture location is proximal metaphyseal or diaphyseal, but distal fractures can also cause delayed swelling and here, too, if a cast has been applied, compartment syndrome is possible. It is important to note that this complication can also occur when the interosseous membrane has been torn, as is the case in more severe fractures, and can even develop in open fractures (5% incidence). The clinical findings of compartment syndrome rely heavily on patient cooperation. Unfortunately, in children this cooperation is frequently not possible, and intracompartmental pressures should be measured in all questionable cases. This is especially relevant for children with head injuries, who are unable to report any symptoms. In such cases, pressures should be obtained routinely. Subsequent monitoring is also indicated if possible increases in tissue pressures are anticipated.

Of the several methods available for measuring intracompartmental pressures, the simplest consists of a hand-held needle pressure sensor (with digital readout). This device can also be attached to a slit catheter for indwelling continuous readings. The pressure threshold for a positive diagnosis may vary somewhat according to the technique used, but for accuracy this reading should be compared with the mean arterial pressure, or, at least, with the diastolic blood pressure. Decompression is recommended when compartment pressures rise to within 20 to 30 mm Hg of the diastolic blood pressure, or if the absolute value is greater than 35 mm Hg. All four compartments should be measured initially.

FIGURE 47
Left, Anteroposterior view of this open tibia fracture with a segmental defect. This was treated with external fixation and a local muscle rotation flap. **Right**, With this type of external fixator, fracture alignment can be easily adjusted through the ball joints in the device.

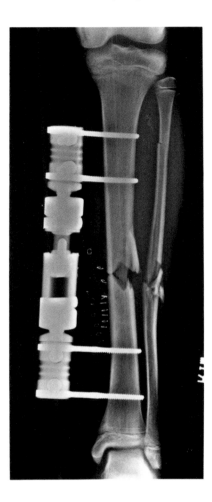 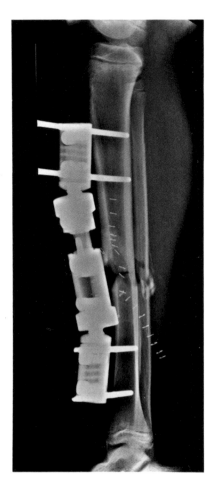

A tense, swollen extremity should alert the physician, especially if there is pain with passive stretching of the muscles in the involved compartment. Any sensory deficit is an absolute sign (decreased light touch or pin prick), unless this finding is a result of a more proximal primary nerve injury. The presence of palpable distal pulses and rapid capillary refill is no assurance that compartmental pressures are not pathologically elevated. Impending syndromes are often first signaled when the child complains of pain that is out of proportion to that expected from the fracture, and this pain is not relieved by the usual amount of mild analgesic medication. The injured leg should not be elevated, because to do so will reduce the mean arterial pressure, causing a subsequent reduction in oxygen perfusion to the compartment and leading to further muscle ischemia, thus perpetuating the syndrome.

Decompression should be performed immediately after diagnosis because the extent

FIGURE 48

Top left and **top center**, Anteroposterior and lateral views of a distal tibia fracture with severe abrasions of the leg and skin loss over the calcaneus. **Top right**, An adult upper extremity external fixator was used to stabilize the fracture, using small pins. **Bottom left**, The frame was extended across the ankle to maintain neutral foot position until the calcaneal wound healed. **Bottom center** and **bottom right**, Final result 12 months later.

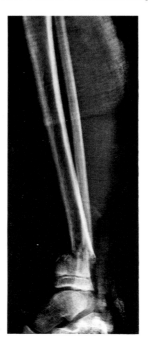
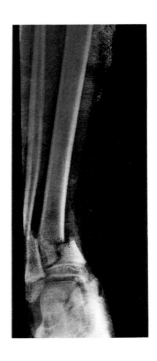
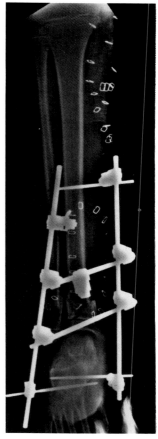
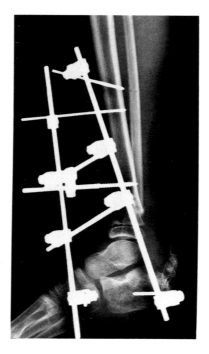
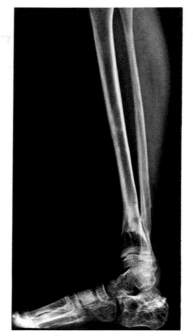
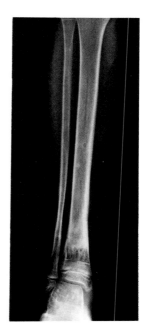

of muscle and nerve damage is time-related. Damage commences as soon as four to six hours after the onset of abnormal pressures. In general, all four compartments should be released, and release is accomplished either through a single lateral incision with complete perifibular dissection, or more routinely through medial and lateral incisions where all vital structures are easily visualized. Fibulectomy is not recommended in children, because it can lead to valgus deformity of the ankle. In those rare cases in which the tibial fracture is complicated by arterial insufficiency, prophylactic four-compartment fasciotomy should be routinely performed in order to prevent a reperfusion compartment syndrome, especially if warm ischemia time has exceeded four hours.

Fasciotomy is generally considered an indication for surgical stabilization of the fractured limb. Stabilization should be accomplished at the time of compartment release, with either internal or external fixation. Rigid stabilization facilitates further wound management, allows for direct continued examination of the extremity, and prevents continued trauma to the soft tissues as the leg is manipulated.

Polytrauma

The child who has sustained multiple fractures and other system injuries is a good candidate for early surgical stabilization of at least all the long-bone fractures. Surgical stabilization greatly facilitates initial intensive care management; improves later patient mobilization, especially in the adolescent; and reduces the length of the hospital stay. In contralateral long-bone fracture of the femur and the tibia, or in bilateral tibia fractures, if one of the injuries has been surgically secured, this extremity will allow earlier weightbearing and greater patient mobility. The special case of ipsilateral femur and tibia fractures will be discussed in the next section.

The head-injured child with multiple fractures in addition to the tibia is also more appropriately managed by surgical intervention. In this instance, external fixation or flexible intramedullary rods can be very effective, and

the avoidance of traction and plaster techniques enhances nursing care.[108]

Floating-Knee Injuries

Ipsilateral fractures of the femur and tibia produce a "floating-knee" configuration. Several different patterns of injury are shown in Figure 49. These fractures are generally high-velocity injuries, and motor vehicle-pedestrian (bicycle rider) collisions are the usual cause of injury. Fracture management can be difficult, because the incidence of complications (nonunion, malunion, knee stiffness, ligamentous derangement, and fat embolism) is high. Current recommendations for adults emphasize an aggressive surgical approach to fixation of both bones.

In children, as in adults, closed treatment can result in a number of problems, especially in adolescents. In fact, Bohn and Durbin[28] found patient age to be the most important variable related to clinical course, noting 10 years of age as the significant divider. In their series, all tibial malunions and significant leg-length discrepancies were in the closed treatment group.

McBryde and Blake[109] reported a 20% rate of delayed union and a 30% rate of malunion in children with floating knees treated by closed management alone. In order to improve on this, Letts and associates[110] recommend that at least one fracture be rigidly fixed in all cases. They cite the tibia as being the most amenable to stabilization. In children, after an external fixator has been placed on the tibia, traction can be applied to treat the femur (Fig. 50). Alternatively, external fixation can be applied to the femur and the tibia casted, if the fracture pattern was stable. However, a long leg cast would have to be placed over the fixator. In adolescents, it is preferable to use internal fixation for the femur at least, because Bohn and Durbin[28] have demonstrated that this treatment is associated with fewer complications and better long-term results.

The indications for surgical stabilization of the tibia are as one might expect: inability to achieve satisfactory closed reduction, open fracture with soft-tissue injury, compartment syndrome, and juxta-articular fracture patterns involving the growth plate. In adolescents ap-

FIGURE 49

Schematic of different floating knee injury patterns, (A) diaphyseal fracture, femur and tibia, (B) diaphyseal and metaphyseal fracture, either bone, (C) physeal and diaphyseal fracture, either bone, (D) one bone open fracture, (E) both bones present as open fractures. (Redrawn with permission from Letts M, Vincent N, Gouw G: The "Floating Knee" in children. *J Bone Joint Surg* 1986;68B:442–446.).

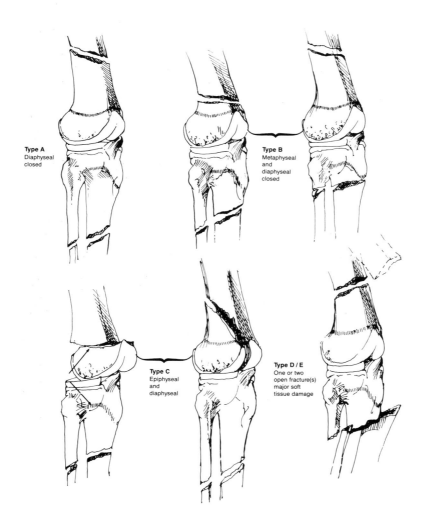

proaching skeletal maturity, the tibia can be stabilized with nonreamed intramedullary rods (see Fig. 51).

One final advantage of the use of rigid stabilization for the floating knee is that it allows a more accurate assessment of knee ligamentous damage (approximately 10% incidence). Rigid stabilization also facilitates further treatment of the knee.

APPLICATION OF EXTERNAL FIXATION DEVICE

Several different types of external fixators are available for the treatment of tibia fractures, ranging from unilateral cantilever systems to circular "ring" fixators. Selection of a particular device is based on the fracture pattern as well as the extent of soft-tissue damage. The more unstable the fracture is, the more

FIGURE 50
In this type D floating knee injury (the tibia
fracture was open), external fixation was
applied to the tibia (**left**), with traction for
the femur (**right**). Casting was eventually
used until the femur healed completely.

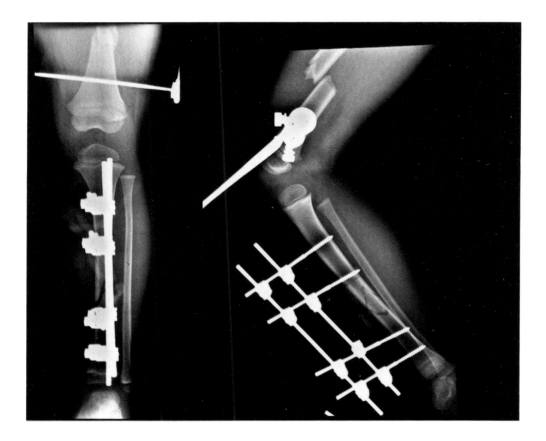

complex the frame construct needs to be (e.g.,
unilateral construct versus triangular frame)
so as to provide increased fracture stability.
Wound access is also important, and the use
of ring fixators is best reserved for later recon-
structive treatment rather than for initial extremity management.

Most cantilever external fixators are applied
to the anteromedial surface of the tibial shaft
and use four half pins for bone fixation. When
possible, pins should not be placed any closer
than 2 cm from the physis, or closer than 2 cm
from the fracture sites. In the case of the tubular fixator, the most distal pin is placed first,
followed by the most proximal pin, with as
much distance between them as possible. The
other two pins are then sequentially placed on
either side of the fracture, as close to it as
possible (Fig. 52). The use of fluoroscopy is
recommended during pin insertion. To en-
hance frame stability, a double bar configuration is generally used and the two bars are
placed as close to the skin as possible, leaving
only enough space to allow for skin care. Fracture reduction should be performed before inserting all four pins, because with this device
malrotation and excessive angulation cannot
be corrected after all the pins are in place.[111]

FIGURE 51
Left, This adolescent has a type B floating knee injury. **Center**, A nonreamed intramedullary tibial nail was used after the femur was fixed internally. **Right**, Six-month follow-up demonstrating tibial healing in good alignment.

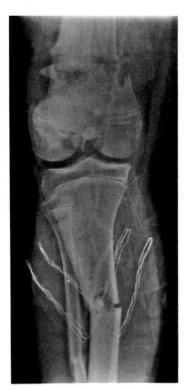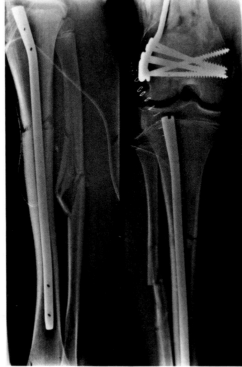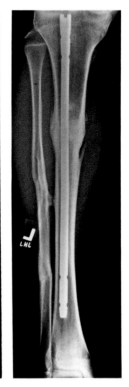

Other external fixators are equipped with universal ball-joints, which allow greater flexibility during application. In this type of fixator, the central body is quite rigid; consequently, pin placement can consist of two pins (one proximal and the other distal to the fracture site) that are widely separated.

Generally, transfixing full pins are not indicated, unless a thin wire, circular fixator is used. In this instance, it is imperative that great attention be paid to cross-sectional anatomy to avoid injury to vital structures during pin insertion. Preassembly of the frame, based on the injury radiographs, expedites application times. With this type of fixator early full weightbearing is encouraged and the fixator can generally remain on the extremity until healing is complete (Fig. 53).

Pin diameter in small children should not exceed 4 mm, but 5- or 6-mm pins can be used for children older than 12 years of age. Occasionally, an external fixator designed for use on the adult upper extremity is an appropriate size to apply to the tibia of a small child.

Pin-tract care involves daily cleansing with cotton applicators moistened with dilute hydrogen peroxide. Antibiotic ointments are not recommended. Once soft-tissue healing is complete, partial to full weightbearing is instituted. The timing for frame removal will depend on evidence of fracture healing, the condition of soft tissue, the quality of pin-tract

FIGURE 52
This demonstrates the pin placement and insertion sequence for the tubular external fixator. **Left**, Insertion of the most distal and then the most proximal screws 2 cm away from the physis. **Center**, The tubular bar is then attached after the remaining adjustable clamps are mounted to the bar. Through these other clamps the next two screws are inserted, staying at least 2 cm from the fracture site. **Right**, A second bar can be applied to increase frame stability. If this is done, the second bar must be connected to the clamps before inserting the third and fourth screws. (Adapted with permission from Alonso JE, Horowitz M: Use of AO/ASIF external fixator in children. *J Pediatr Orthop* 1987;7:596.)

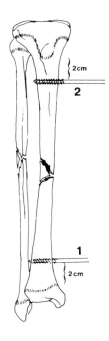 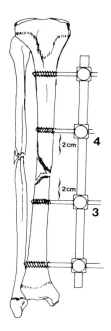 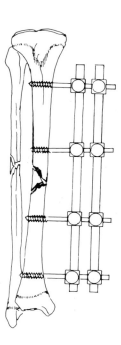

care, and the preference of the treating surgeon.

 ANKLE FRACTURES

GENERAL CONSIDERATIONS

Anatomy

The anatomy of the ankle in children is like that of the adult, except for the physes and their growth. As in the adult, the ankle is a hinge (ginglymus) joint comprised of the tibia, fibula, and talus. The deltoid ligament arises from the medial malleolus and separates into two parts; the deep portion, which inserts into the medial talus, and the superficial portion, which attaches to the navicular, talus, and calcaneus (sustentacular tali). The lateral ligamentous complex consists of three individual ligaments: anterior talofibular, posterior talofibular, and calcaneofibular. Both the medial and the lateral ligaments arise from the tibia and fibula distal to the physis. The syndesmosis consists of the anterior and posterior tibiofibular ligaments and the distal portion of the interosseous ligament. The anterior tibiofibular ligament also arises distal to the physis.

The distal tibial epiphysis (secondary ossification center) usually becomes visible on radiographs during the first year.[112] Initially, the physis is transverse, but within two years

FIGURE 53
Top left, Grade II open tibia fracture in a 12-year-old child. **Top center** and **top right**, Treatment with circular external fixator, anteroposterior and lateral views.

Bottom left, Full weightbearing was possible, until complete healing 3 months later (**bottom right**).

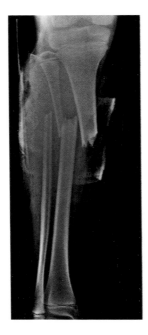
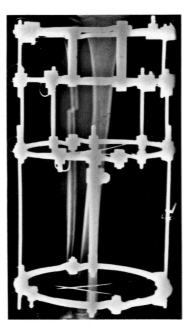
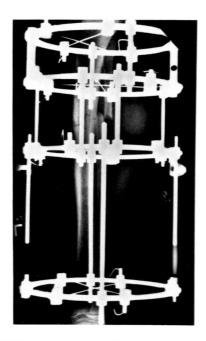
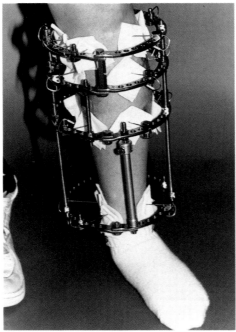
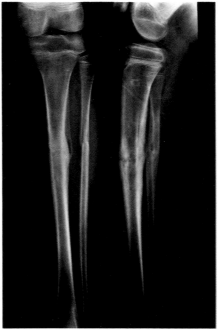

FIGURE 54
Diagrammatic illustration of physeal injuries involving the distal tibia and fibula. 1 = supination-inversion, 2 = pronation-eversion-external rotation, 3 = supination-plantar flexion, 4 = supination-external rotation. With the supination-external rotation and supination-inversion mechanisms, stage I indicates that only the tibia is fractured and stage II indicates that both the tibia and fibula are fractured. (Reproduced with permission from Dias LS: Fractures of the tibia and fibula, in Rockwood CA Jr, Wilkins KE, King RE (eds): *Fractures in Children.* Philadelphia, JB Lippincott, 1984, p 1016.)

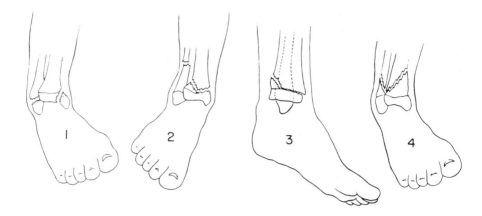

an anteromedial undulation develops, which separates the distal tibial epiphysis into medial and lateral regions. Ossification of the medial malleolus begins from this center and occurs at around seven years of age in girls and eight years in boys. Eventually, the entire distal tibial epiphysis and medial malleolus become ossified and fuse with the metaphysis. This physiologic epiphysiodesis occurs between the ages of 12 and 14 years in girls and 15 and 18 years in boys. Closure starts centrally, then medially, and finally proceeds laterally;[113] usually this closure occurs over an 18-month time span.

The distal fibular epiphysis appears by two to three years of age. However, its epiphysiodesis with the metaphysis occurs later than that of the tibia, at approximately 19 to 20 years of age.

Mechanism of Injury

In children, ankle fractures nearly always involve the distal tibial and fibular epiphyseal plates, and these fractures usually occur by indirect mechanisms. Dias and Tachdjian[114] have combined the Salter-Harris anatomic scheme

OUTLINE 3
Classification of distal tibial and fibular physeal fractures

I. Supination—external rotation (SER)
   a. Stage I
   b. Stage II
II. Pronation-eversion-external rotation (PEER)
III. Supination-plantar flexion (SPF)
IV. Supination-inversion (SI)
   a. Stage I
   b. Stage II
V. Axial compression
VI. Juvenile Tillaux
VII. Triplane fractures
VIII. Other physeal injuries

(Reproduced with permission from Dias LS: Fractures of the tibia and fibula, in Rockwood CA Jr, Wilkins KE, King RE (eds): *Fractures in Children.* Philadelphia, JB Lippincott, 1984, vol III, p 1016.)

with the Lauge-Hansen mechanistic scheme (Outline 3 and Fig. 54).[78,115] In this classification, the foot is fixed in the first named po-

FIGURE 55

A three-dimensional reconstruction of a triplane fracture. The computer software subtracted out the fibula, leaving only a view of the distal tibia. Note the Tillaux component (white arrow) as well as an incidental, nondisplaced, previously undiagnosed medial malleolus vertical shear fracture (black arrow). **Top left,** The anteroposterior radiograph. **Top right,** The lateral radiograph. **Bottom,** The three-dimensional reconstruction.

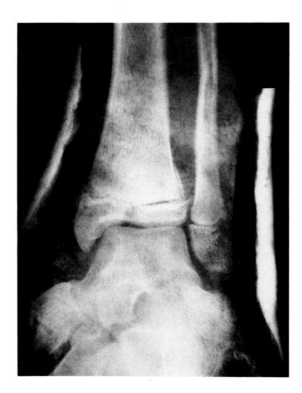
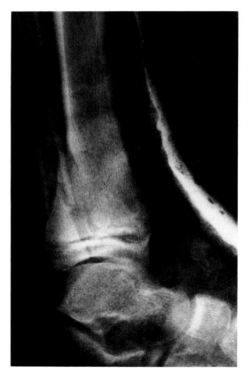
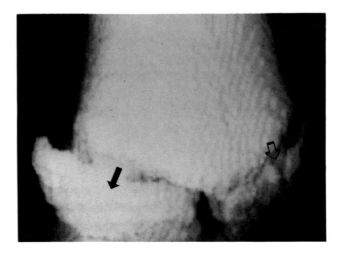

sition and the leg moves over the foot in the second named direction. This classification is useful during closed reductions, in which the direction of the abnormal force is reversed, and the foot and ankle are immobilized in the position opposite to that of the mechanism of fracture.

Evaluation

After a closed reduction, standard anteroposterior, lateral, and mortise radiographs are reviewed. It is often difficult to assess the magnitude of joint incongruity or fracture displacement on plain radiographs. If there is any question, further studies should be performed using either a computed tomographic scan or tomograms. The computed tomographic scan can give excellent visualization through plaster casts, and fracture displacement can be measured electronically on the computer image.[116,117]

Sagittal and coronal plane reconstructions from the computed tomographic scan easily demonstrate joint congruity. In comminuted fractures, mental reconstruction of the computed tomographic scan in the surgeon's mind can be difficult. If three-dimensional reconstruction is available, it can be used to visualize the fracture patterns (Fig. 55). The computed tomographic scan can be helpful in planning incision placement.

Surgical Indications

If the standard radiographs and/or computed tomographic scan or tomograms do not show acceptable alignment, then surgery is indicated. Generally, all Salter types I and II fractures can be treated closed. Open reduction is required only if there is soft-tissue interposition (usually periosteum) that prevents reduction, or if there is an unacceptable valgus or varus deformity.

The amount of angulation that is acceptable decreases with the older child, because less remodeling can occur. In children older than 12 or 13 years of age, deformity can no longer be expected to remodel.[118] Even in the young child, valgus angulation greater than 15 to 20 degrees will not correct with remodeling and should be surgically reduced.[119] As the child matures, the growth remaining in the distal

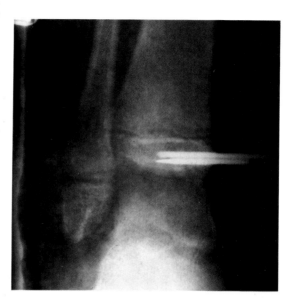

FIGURE 56

An anteroposterior radiograph of a Salter IV medial malleolus fracture after open reduction/internal fixation with smooth transepiphyseal K-wires.

tibial epiphysis cannot compensate for angulation, and adult criteria should be used (5 degrees of varus or valgus and 5 to 10 degrees of anterior or posterior angulation). This change occurs at approximately 10 years of age for girls and 11 years for boys.[120]

Salter types III and IV fractures require accurate anatomic reduction to minimize the risk of premature growth arrest,[121] to align the joint surfaces, and to restore the ankle mortise. Any joint incongruity or displacement greater than 2 mm is unacceptable and requires surgical reduction and fixation.

Techniques of Open Reduction/Internal Fixation

In those fractures where only soft-tissue interposition is present, open reduction and removal of the interposed tissues is usually sufficient to permit a stable reduction of the fragment, which can then be held by cast immobilization alone. If fragments are not stable, internal fixation should be used. If at all possible, the fixation device should not cross the

FIGURE 57
Left, A Salter III medial malleolus fracture at the time of injury in a child 8 years and 1 month of age. The fracture was treated nonoperatively. **Right**, A growth deformity comprised of a physeal bar (arrow) and articular joint malunion occurred as seen in the tomogram at age 9 years and 2 months.

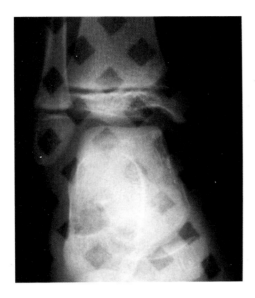
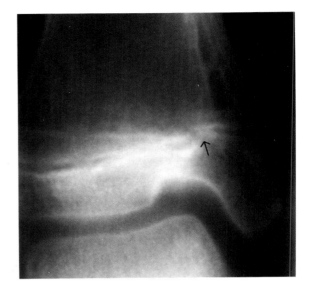

physis. Techniques that can be used if the fracture is a Salter type II are transmetaphyseal screws that fix the Thurston-Holland fragment to the remaining metaphysis without violating the physis.

For the very rare Salter type I fracture that remains unstable after the interposed soft-tissue has been removed, fixation can sometimes be maintained by resuturing the avulsed metaphyseal periosteum back to its origin, either through drill holes in bone (with absorbable suture) or to the other periosteal margin. If this does not work, then one or two small, smooth K-wires that pass from the epiphysis into the metaphysis can be used. To minimize physeal trauma, multiple passes of the wire should be avoided. The wires should be removed as soon as the fracture is stable (usually three to six weeks). This fixation should be supplemented with a short or long leg cast, depending on the intraoperative stability. Whether fixation has been used or not, final intraoperative radiographs should be obtained before wound closure.

Again, for Salter types III and IV fractures, the fixation devices should not cross the physis unless it is already undergoing the final stage of physiologic epiphysiodesis (e.g., juvenile Tillaux fractures). Transepiphyseal and/or transmetaphyseal fixation, using screws or wires that transfix the two epiphyseal or metaphyseal fragments and parallel the physis, is preferred (Fig. 56).

SPECIFIC ANKLE FRACTURES

Medial Malleolus

Fractures of the medial malleolus are usually Salter types III or IV and often occur in young children.[60,115,118,120] The articular surface must be anatomically reduced. These fractures also have a high incidence of growth arrest and osseous bridging.[121]

Closed treatment should be used only in fractures that are clearly not displaced, and even then, close and frequent follow-up is required to insure that proximal migration or rotation with malunion and osseous bridging does not develop (Fig. 57). For these reasons,

FIGURE 58
Radiographs of a juvenile Tillaux fracture. Although the fracture (arrow) can be seen on the anteroposterior radiograph (**top left**), it is much clearer on the mortise radiograph (**top right**). It was treated by anatomic open reduction and internal fixation (**bottom**).

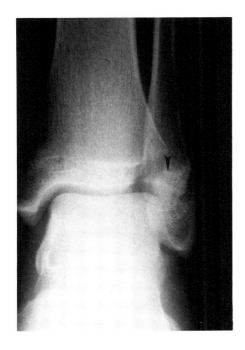
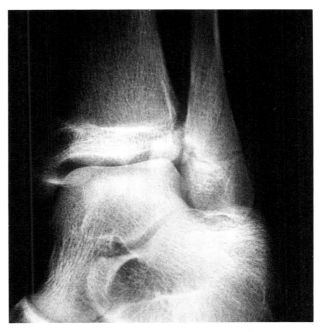
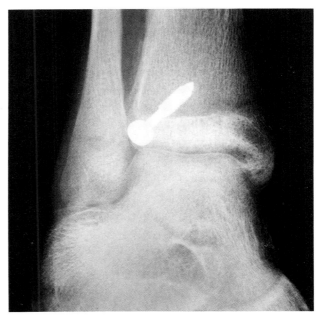

FIGURE 59
The three fragments of a three-part triplane fracture: (1) anterolateral portion of the distal tibial epiphysis, (2) remainder of the epiphysis with an attached posteromedial spike of the distal tibial metaphysis, (3) the remainder of the distal tibial metaphysis. (Reproduced with permission from Dias LS: Fractures of the tibia and fibula, in Rockwood CA Jr, Wilkins KE, King RE (eds): *Fractures in Children.* Philadelphia, JB Lippincott, 1984, p 1023.)

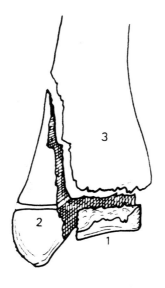 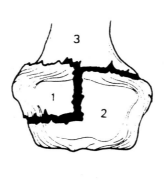

young patients with distal tibial physeal fractures should be carefully assessed to ensure that the fracture is reduced in all planes. If there is any doubt regarding the ability to achieve and maintain satisfactory closed reduction, an open reduction should be performed, and the anatomic reduction maintained with smooth K-wires. The wires must not traverse the physis but, rather, must parallel it. Small metaphyseal screws can also be used—the newer small cannulated screws will facilitate this method.

Transitional Fractures

Transitional fractures are those that occur during physiologic epiphysiodesis of the distal tibial physis. The two main types of transitional fracture are the triplane fracture and the juvenile Tillaux. With these fractures, the potential for growth deformities is low, because they occur near skeletal maturity.[122] Ankle joint congruity, not growth deformity, is now the major concern.

Juvenile Tillaux The juvenile Tillaux fracture, a Salter type III fracture of the anterolateral distal tibial epiphysis, is caused by an external rotation force and avulsion of the Salter III fragment by the anterior tibiofibular ligament.[119] The mortise and lateral views are very useful in recognizing and assessing fracture displacement.[123] Any ambiguity should be further explored with a computed tomographic scan. No more than 2 mm of displacement should be accepted. Either screw or pin fixation can be used, and fixation can now cross the physis (Fig. 58), because the remaining growth potential is minimal.

Triplane Fractures In triplane fractures, the fracture line involves the transverse, sagittal, and coronal planes to create Salter types III and IV injuries.[124] The displaced fragments may be either medial or lateral (external rotation mechanism) and may consist of two,[124] three,[125] and occasionally four parts (Fig.

FIGURE 60

An example of a triplane fracture in a 14-year-old boy treated by open reduction and internal fixation. **Top left,** The anteroposterior radiograph. **Top right,** The lateral radiograph. **Center left,** The computed tomographic scan cut above the level of the physis shows the posteromedial metaphyseal spike (single arrow) (part 3) and **(center right)** the cut just below the physis shows the juvenile Tillaux component (double arrow) (part 1). **Bottom left** and **bottom right,** The computed tomographic scan cut at the level of the medial malleolus shows an unexpected minimally displaced vertical shear fracture through the medial malleolus (single arrow; TD-talar dome). Because of the anterolateral Tillaux, the posteromedial metaphyseal spike, and medial malleolus fractures, the open reduction and internal fixation was performed through two exposures: anterolateral and posteromedial.

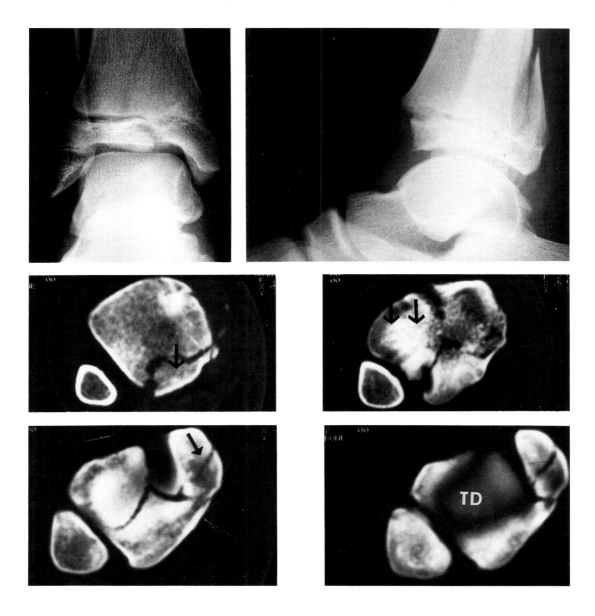

FIGURE 61

Left, Same patient as Figure 60. Anteroposterior and lateral radiographs **(right)** six weeks after open reduction internal fixation. The Tillaux component was fixed with smooth pins crossing the physis.

Pins (rather than screws) were elected because, although the chronologic age was 14 years, the bone age was 12 years.

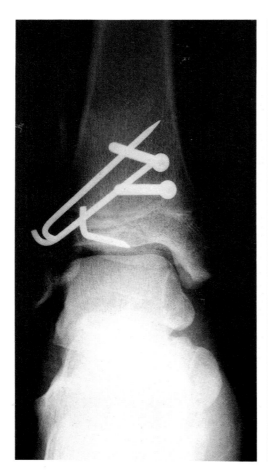
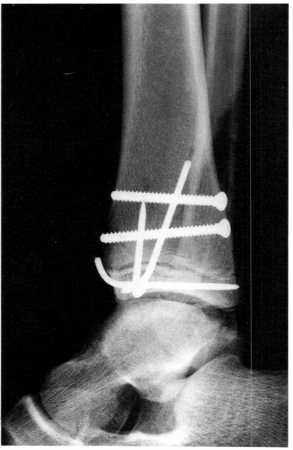

59).[117] An open reduction should be done if there is 2 mm or more separation or displacement at the fracture site.

With triplane fractures, the computed tomographic scan can be very useful in (1) identifying the exact anatomy and (2) planning the surgical incisions (Figs. 60 and 61). Usually two incisions are required.

At the time of surgery, the fragments are debrided of all loose material, the joint is thoroughly irrigated, and anatomic reduction is performed. There is often periosteal interposition at the juvenile Tillaux component of the triplane. After anatomic reduction, the fracture is internally fixed. Fixation both above and below the physis is often necessary (especially for three and four part fractures). In general, interfragmentary screws are preferable to wires, because they allow compression of the fracture fragments.

FIGURE 62

This 6-year-old boy sustained a severe lawn mower injury to his hind foot. The Achilles tendon had a 1.5-cm substance loss. There was also a large transverse laceration ("Cincinnati incision" type), along with an open calcaneus fracture **(left)**. Irrigation and debridement was done four times at 48- to 72-hour intervals. At the last debridement, the calcaneus was reduced and internally fixed with three K-wires **(right)**. The wound healed by both delayed primary closure and secondary intention. A delayed reconstruction of the heel cord was performed approximately 10 weeks after injury. There has never been any sign of sepsis.

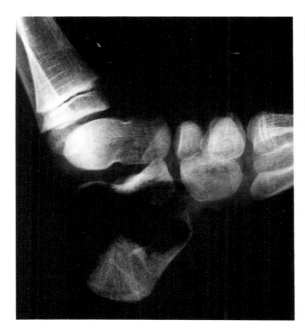
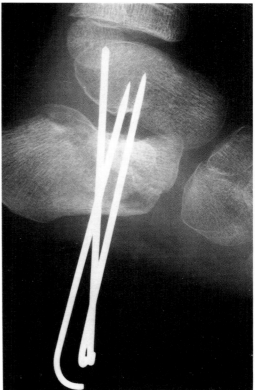

 FOOT FRACTURES

GENERAL CONSIDERATIONS

Fractures of the foot in children are rare and it is even rarer for such a fracture to require surgical treatment. Fractures that do require surgical treatment are nearly always the result of severe trauma, and they often involve open injuries that are associated with soft-tissue management problems.

The calcaneus is the most commonly fractured tarsal bone in children. These fractures are often open ones, such as are seen with lawn mower or boat propeller injuries. With these open injuries, the initial treatment must

FIGURE 63

This 12-year-old boy sustained a comminuted calcaneus fracture, as shown in the lateral (**top**) and axial (**bottom left**) views. A computed tomographic scan (**bottom right**) delineates the two major fragments, the medial sustentacular fragment (S) and the tuberosity fragment (T). The tuberosity fragment is compressed and pushed laterally, disrupting the subtalar joint.

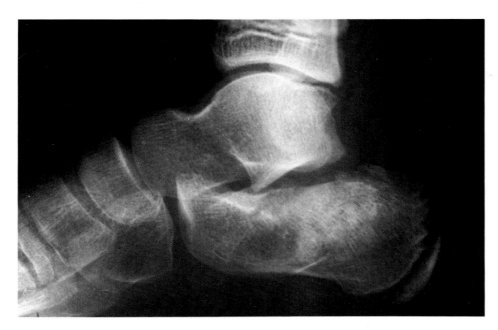

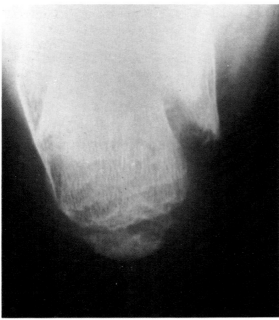

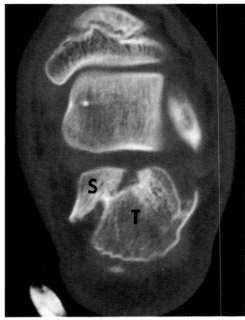

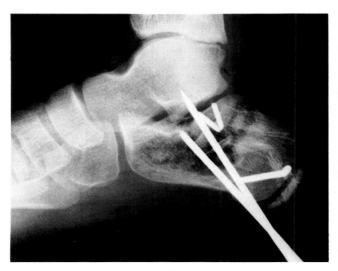
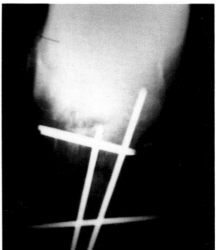

be concerned primarily with the soft tissues and with obtaining adequate irrigation and debridement. Splints should be used rather than casts for these injuries, and multiple debridements (every 24 to 48 hours) are necessary. Occasionally, bone stabilization is required, with either internal or external fixation, and soft-tissue reconstruction is often necessary (Fig. 62).

In adolescents, calcaneus fractures frequently parallel those of the adult with regard to mechanism of injury (falls from heights), fracture patterns (e.g., subtalar joint involvement, decreases in Böhler's angle), and treatment. In children older than 10 or 11 years of age, the calcaneal anatomy is like that of an adult, and minimal remodeling potential is present. In these circumstances, assessment of intra-articular involvement of fracture displacement should be done with tomograms or computed tomographic scan as in an adult.[126] Open reduction and internal fixation should be considered (Figs. 63 and 64).

The talus is rarely fractured, unless it is run over by a car or injured by open trauma, as in a lawn mower accident. When severe closed injuries occur, it is usually in the older child and here, as in the calcaneus, injuries tend to parallel those of the adult with regard to fracture pattern (talar neck) and treatment. Open reduction and internal fixation is rarely required for pediatric talus fractures.

Indications for open reduction of talar neck fractures in children parallel those of the adult,[125] where displacement must be less than 5 mm and malalignment less than 5 degrees on the anteroposterior view.[127] There is controversy regarding the best approach for open reduction. Some authors recommend a dorsal-medial approach between the extensor hallucis longus and anterior tibial tendons.[128] Others recommend a lateral approach.[60] No matter which approach is used, the surgical exposure should lessen the risk of osteonecrosis by avoiding extensive dissection. Less harm will be done by accepting minor displacement (with either closed or open treatment) than will occur with repeated closed reductions or extensive soft-tissue dissection performed in an attempt to achieve a truly anatomic open reduction.

FIGURE 65
This 10-year-old girl sustained a severe gunshot wound to her foot (**left**) which was treated with multiple irrigations and debridements. The multiple open metatarsal fractures with bony loss were stabilized by multiple K-wires (**right**). (Reproduced with permission from Stucky WS, Loder RT: Extremity gunshot wounds in children. *J Pediatr Orthop* 1991;11:64–71.)

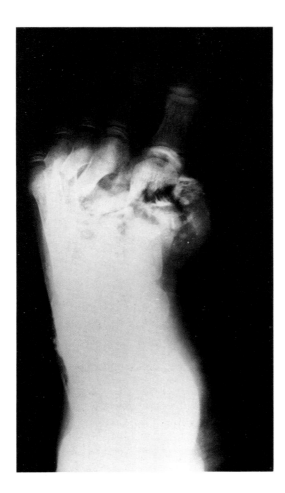
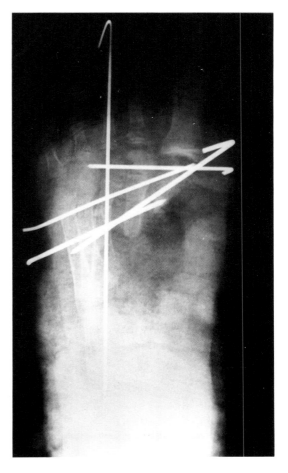

The means of fixation of talar neck fractures can either be multiple K-wires, or screws, if the talus is large enough to accommodate them. If osteonecrosis develops, revascularization in children is usually more complete than it is in adults.[129]

Injuries to the metatarsals, although they are relatively common in children, rarely require surgical treatment. The exception is for open injuries, as from lawn mowers. Here again, the main emphasis should be placed on adequate debridement and early soft-tissue coverage.

The metatarsals can be easily internally or externally fixed with multiple smooth K-wires (Fig. 65), and they should be splinted rather than stabilized with a circumferential cast. Multiple debridements and dressing changes in the operating room should be continued until the wounds are clean and show signs of good granulation tissue.

REFERENCES

1. Eichelberger MR, Mangubat EA, Sacco WJ, et al: Outcome analysis of blunt injury in children. *J Trauma* 1988;28:1109–1117.

2. Gratz RR: Accidental injury in childhood: A literature review on pediatric trauma. *J Trauma* 1979;19:551–555.

3. Marcus RE, Mills MF, Thompson GH: Multiple injury in children. *J Bone Joint Surg* 1983;65A:1291–1294.

4. Lange RH, Bach AW, Hansen ST Jr, et al: Open tibial fractures with associated vascular injuries: Prognosis for limb salvage. *J Trauma* 1985;25:203–208.

5. Ziv I, Rang M: Treatment of femoral fracture in the child with head injury. *J Bone Joint Surg* 1983;65B:276–278.

6. Wagner MB, McCabe JB: A comparison of four techniques to establish intraosseous infusion. *Pediatr Emerg Care* 1988;4:87–91.

7. Hahn YS, Chyung C, Barthel MJ, et al: Head injuries in children under 36 months of age: Demography and outcome. *Child's Nerv Syst* 1988;4:34–40.

8. Anderson WA: The significance of femoral fractures in children. *Ann Emerg Med* 1982;11:174–177.

9. Barlow B, Niemirska M, Gandhi R, et al: Response to injury in children with closed femur fractures. *J Trauma* 1987;27:429–430.

10. Tepas JJ III, Ramenofsky ML, Mollitt DL, et al: The pediatric trauma score as a predictor of injury severity: An objective assessment. *J Trauma* 1988;28:425–529.

11. Kaufmann CR, Maier RV, Rivara FP, et al: Evaluation of the pediatric trauma score. *JAMA* 1990;263:69–72.

12. Reilly PL, Simpson DA, Sprod R, et al: Assessing the conscious level in infants and young children: A paediatric version of the Glasgow Coma Scale. *Child's Nerv Syst* 1988;4:30–33.

13. Loder RT: Pediatric polytrauma: Orthopaedic care and hospital course. *J Orthop Trauma* 1987;1:48–54.

14. Love SM, Grogan DP, Ogden JA: Lawn-mower injuries in children. *J Orthop Trauma* 1988;2:94–101.

15. Bachulis BL, Long WB, Hynes GD, et al: Clinical indications for cervical spine radiographs in the traumatized patient. *Am J Surg* 1987;153:473–477.

16. Shaffer MA, Doris PE: Limitation of the cross table lateral view in detecting cervical spine injuries: A retrospective review. *Am Emerg Med* 1981;10:508–513.

17. Rachesky I, Boyce WT, Duncan B, et al: Clinical prediction of cervical spine injuries in children: Radiographic abnormalities. *Am J Dis Child* 1987;141:199–201.

18. Hadden WA, Gillespie WJ: Multiple level injuries of the cervical spine. *Injury* 1985;16:628–633.

19. Acheson MB, Livingston RR, Richardson ML, et al: High-resolution CT scanning in the evaluation of cervical spine fractures: Comparison with plain film examinations. *Am J Radiol* 1987;148:1179–1185.

20. Herzenberg JE, Hensinger RN, Dedrick DK, et al: Emergency transport and positioning of young children who have an injury to the cervical spine: The standard back board may be hazardous. *J Bone Joint Surg* 1989;71A:15–22.

21. Bach A, Johansen K: Limb salvage using temporary arterial shunt following traumatic near-amputation of the thigh. *J Pediatr Orthop* 1982;2:187–190.

22. Riseborough EJ, Barrett IR, Shapiro F: Growth disturbances following distal femoral physeal fracture-separations. *J Bone Joint Surg* 1983;65A:885–893.

23. Spiegel PG, Mast JW: Internal and external fixation of fractures in children. *Orthop Clin North Am* 1980;11:405–421.

24. Rang ML: *The Growth Plate and Its Disorders.* Edinburgh, E & S Livingstone Ltd., 1969.

25. Ogden JA: Skeletal growth mechanism injury patterns. *J Pediat Orthop* 1982;2:371–377.

26. Buckley SL, Smith G, Sponseller PD, et al: Open fractures of the tibia in children. *J Bone Joint Surg* 1990;72A:1462–1469.

27. Hoffer MM, Garrett A, Brink J, et al: The orthopaedic management of brain-injured children. *J Bone Joint Surg* 1971;53A:567–577.

28. Bohn WW, Durbin RA: Ipsilateral fractures of the femur and tibia in children and adolescents. *J Bone Joint Surg* 1991;73A:429–439.

29. Garvin KL, McCarthy RE, Barnes CL, et al: Pediatric pelvic ring fractures. *J Pediatr Orthop* 1990;10:577–582.

30. Reff RB: The use of external fixation devices in the management of severe lower-extremity trauma and pelvic injuries in children. *Clin Orthop* 1984;188:21–33.

31. Nakayama DK, Ramenofsky ML, Rowe MI: Chest injuries in childhood. *Am Surg* 1989;210:770–775.

32. Stanford JR, Evans WE, Morse TS: Pediatric arterial injuries. *J Vasc Dis* 1976;27:1–7.

33. Friedman RJ, Jupiter JB: Vascular injuries and closed extremity fractures in children. *Clin Orthop* 1984;188:112–119.

34. Green NE, Allen BL: Vascular injuries associated with dislocation of the knee. *J Bone Joint Surg* 1977;59A:236–239.

35. Navarre JR, Cardillo PJ, Gorman JF, et al: Vascular trauma in children and adolescents. *Am J Surg* 1982;143:229–231.

36. Smith PL, Lim WN, Ferris EJ, et al: Emergency arteriography in extremity trauma: Assessment of indications: *Am J Roentgenol* 1981;137:803–807.

37. Russo VJ: Case Report: Traumatic arterial spasm resulting in gangrene. *J Pediatr Orthop* 1985;5:486–488.

38. Samson R, Pasternak BM: Traumatic arterial spasm—rarity or nonentity. *J Trauma* 1980;20:607–609.

39. Fabian TC, Turkleson ML, Connelly TL, et al: Injury to the popliteal artery. *Am J Surg* 1982;143:225–228.

40. Kirby RM, Winquist RA, Hansen ST: Femoral shaft fractures in adolescents: A comparison between traction plus cast treatment and closed intramedullary nailing. *J Pediatr Orthop* 1981;1:193–197.

41. Henard DC, Bobo RT: Avulsion fractures of the tibial tubercle in adolescents: A report of bilateral fractures and a review of the literature. *Clin Orthop* 1983;177:182–187.

42. Thompson GH, Wilber JH, Marcus RE: Internal fixation of fractures in children and adolescents: A comparative analysis. *Clin Orthop* 1984;188:10–20.

43. Goodrich A, Major MC, Ballard A: Posterior cruciate ligament avulsion associated with ipsilateral femur fracture in a 10-year-old child. *J Trauma* 1988;28:1393–1396.

44. Herndon WA, Mahnken RF, Yngve DA, et al: Management of femoral shaft fractures in the adolescent. *J Pediatr Orthop* 1989;9:29–32.

45. Ziv I, Blackburn N, Rang M: Femoral intramedullary nailing in the growing child. *J Trauma* 1984;24:432–434.

46. Tolo VT: External skeletal fixation in children's fractures. *J Pediatr Orthop* 1983;3:435–442.

47. Ratliff AHC: Fractures of the neck of the femur in children. *J Bone Joint Surg* 1962;44B:528–542.

48. Canale ST, Bourland WL: Fracture of the neck and intertrochanteric region of the femur in children. *J Bone Joint Surg* 1977;59A:431–443.

49. Colonna PC: Fractures of the neck of the femur in children. *Am J Surg* 1929;6:793.

50. Canale ST, King RE: Pelvic and hip fractures, in Rockwood CA Jr, Wilkins KE, King RE (eds): *Fractures in Children*. Philadelphia, JB Lippincott, 1984, chap 9, pp 733–843.

51. Ingram AJ, Bachynski B: Fractures of the hip in children: Treatment and results. *J Bone Joint Surg* 1953;35A:867–887.

52. Lam SF: Fractures of the neck of the femur in children: *J Bone Joint Surg* 1971;53A:1165–1179.

53. Leung PC, Lam SF: Long-term follow-up of children with femoral neck fractures. *J Bone Joint Surg* 1986;68B:537–540.

54. Pforringer W, Rosemeyer B: Fractures of the hip in children and adolescents. *Acta Orthop Scand* 1980;51:91–108.

55. Ratliff AHC: Fractures of the neck of the femur in children. *Orthop Clin North Am* 1974;5:903–923.

56. Swiontkowski MF, Winquist RA: Displaced hip fractures in children and adolescents. *J Trauma* 1986;26:384–388.

57. Edgren W: Coxa plana: A clinical and radiological investigation with particular reference to the importance of the metaphyseal changes for the final shape of the proximal part of the femur. *Acta Ortop Scand* 1965;84(suppl):1–129.

58. Trueta J: The normal vascular anatomy of the human femoral head during growth. *J Bone Joint Surg* 1957;39B:358–394.

59. Chung SMK: The arterial supply of the developing proximal end of the human femur. *J Bone Joint Surg* 1976;58A:961–970.

60. Ogden JA: *Skeletal Injury in the Child*, ed 2. Philadelphia, WB Saunders, 1990.

61. Bucholz RW, Ezaki M, Ogden JA: Injury to the acetabular triradiate physeal cartilage. *J Bone Joint Surg* 1982;64A:600–609.

62. Heeg M, Klasen HJ, Visser JD: Acetabular fractures in children and adolescents. *J Bone Joint Surg* 1989;71B:418–421.

63. Torode I, Zieg D: Pelvic fractures in children. *J Pediatr Orthop* 1985;5:76–84.

64. Heeg M, Viser JD, Oostvogel HJM: Injuries of the acetabular triradiate cartilage and sacroiliac joint. *J Bone Joint Surg* 1988;70B:34–37.

65. Scuderi G, Bronson MJ: Triradiate cartilage injury: Report of two cases and review of the literature. *Clin Orthop* 1987;217:179–189.

66. Blount W: *Fractures in Children*. Baltimore, William & Wilkins, 1955.

67. Hresko MT, Kasser JR: Physeal arrest about the knee associated with nonphyseal fractures in the lower extremity. *J Bone Joint Surg* 1989;71A:698–703.

68. Brouwer KJ, Molenaar JC, van Linge B: Rotational deformities after femoral fractures in childhood: A retrospective study 27–32 years after the accident. *Acta Orthop Scand* 1981;52:81–89.

69. Allen BL Jr, Kant AP, Emery FE: Displaced fractures of the femoral diaphysis in children: Definitive treatment in a double spica cast. *J Trauma* 1977;17:8–19.

70. Staheli LT, Sheridan GW: Early spica cast management of femoral shaft fractures in young children. *Clin Orthop* 1977;126:162–166.

71. Lichtman HM, Duffy J: Lower-extremity balanced traction: A modification of Russell Traction. *Clin Orthop* 1969;66:144–147.

72. Miller PR, Welch MC: The hazards of tibial pin replacement in 90–90 skeletal traction. *Clin Orthop* 1978;135:97–100.

73. Clanton TO, DeLee JC, Sanders B, et al: Knee ligament injuries in children. *J Bone Joint Surg* 1979;61A:1195–1201.

74. Ogden S: *Skeletal Injury in the Child.* Philadelphia, WB Saunders, 1990, chap 19, pp 787–790.

75. Mann DC, Rajmaira S: Distribution of physeal and nonphyseal fractures in 2,650 long-bone fractures in children aged 0–16 years. *J Pediatr Orthop* 1990;10:713–716.

76. Peterson CA, Peterson HA: Analysis of the incidence of injuries to the epiphyseal growth plate. *J Trauma* 1972;12:275–281.

77. Bhaduri T: Meniscectomy in children. *Injury* 1972;3:176–178.

78. Salter RB, Harris WR: Injuries involving the epiphyseal plate. *J Bone Joint Surg* 1963;45A:587–622.

79. Meyers MH: Isolated avulsion of the tibial attachment of the posterior cruciate ligament of the knee. *J Bone Joint Surg* 1975;57A:669–672.

80. Meyers MH, McKeever FM: Fracture of the intercondylar eminence of the tibia. *J Bone Joint Surg* 1970;52A:1677–1684.

81. Meyers MH, McKeever FM: Fractures of the intercondylar eminence of the tibia. *J Bone Joint Surg* 1959;41A:209–215.

82. Zaricznyj B: Avulsion fracture of the tibial eminence: Treatment by open reduction and pinning. *J Bone Joint Surg* 1977;59A:1111–1114.

83. Ross AC, Chesterman PJ: Brief report: Isolated avulsion of the tibial attachment of the posterior cruciate ligament in childhood. *J Bone Joint Surg* 1986;68B:747.

84. Sanders WE, Wilkins KE, Neidre A: Acute insufficiency of the posterior cruciate ligament in children: Two case reports. *J Bone Joint Surg* 1980;62A:129–131.

85. Brunner C: Fracture in and around the knee joint in children and adolescents, in Weber BG, Brunner C, Freuler F (eds): *Treatment of Fractures in Children and Adolescents.* New York, Springer Verlag, 1979, pp 294–323.

86. Bolesta MJ, Fitch RD: Tibial tubercle avulsions. *J Pediatr Orthop* 1986;6:186–192.

87. Ogden JA, Tross RB, Murphy MJ: Fractures of the tibial tuberosity in adolescents. *J Bone Joint Surg* 1980;62A:205–215.

88. Aitken AP: Fractures of the proximal tibial epiphysial cartilage. *Clin Orthop* 1965;41:92–97.

89. Aitken AP, Ingersoll RE: Fractures of the proximal tibial epiphysis. *J Bone Joint Surg* 1956;38A:787–796.

90. Burkhart SS, Peterson HA: Fractures of the proximal tibial epiphysis. *J Bone Joint Surg* 1979;61A:996–1002.

91. Shelton WR, Canale ST: Fractures of the tibia through the proximal tibial epiphyseal cartilage. *J Bone Joint Surg* 1979;61A:167–173.

92. Thompson GH, Gesler JW: Proximal tibial epiphyseal fracture in an infant. *J Pediatr Orthop* 1984;4:114–117.

93. Ahstrom JP: Osteochondral fracture in the knee joint associated with hypermobility and dislocation of the patella: Report of eighteen cases. *J Bone Joint Surg* 1965;47A:1491–1502.

94. Harmon PH: Intra-articular osteochondral fracture as a cause for internal derangement of the knee in adolescents. *J Bone Joint Surg* 1945;27A:703–705.

95. Rosenberg NJ: Osteochondral fractures of the lateral femoral condyle. *J Bone Joint Surg* 1962;46A:1013–1026.

96. van Holsbeeck M, Vandamme B, Marchal G, et al: Dorsal defect of the patella: Concept of its origin and relationship with bipartite and multipartite patella. *Skeletal Radiol* 1987;16:304–311.

97. Ogden JA, McCarthy SM, Jokl P: The painful bipartite patella. *J Pediatr Orthop* 1982;2:263–269.

98. Peterson L, Stener B: Distal disinertion of the patellar ligament combined with avulsion fractures at the medial and lateral margins of the patella: A case report and an experimental study. *Acta Orthop Scand* 1976;47:680–685.

99. Houghton GR, Ackroyd CE: Sleeve fractures of the patella in children: A report of three cases. *J Bone Joint Surg* 1979;61B:65–168.

100. Ogden JA: *Skeletal Injury in the Children.* Philadelphia, Lea & Febiger, 1982, pp 587–592.

101. Jordan SE, Alonso JE, Cook FF: The etiology of valgus angulation after metaphyseal frac-

tures of the tibia in children. *J Pediatr Orthop* 1987;7:450–457.

102. Robert M, Khouri N, Carlioz H, et al: Fractures of the proximal tibial metaphysis in children. *J Pediatr Orthop* 1987;7:444–449.

103. Salter RB, Best T: The pathogenesis and prevention of valgus deformity following fractures of the proximal metaphyseal region of the tibia in children. *J Bone Joint Surg* 1973;55A:1324.

104. Zionts LE, MacEwen GD: Spontaneous improvement of post-traumatic tibia valga. *J Bone Joint Surg* 1986;68A:680–687.

105. Wood D, Hoffer MM: Tibial fractures in head-injured children. *J Trauma* 1987;27:65–68.

106. Shannak AO: Tibial fractures in children: Follow-up study. *J Pediatr Orthop* 1988;8:306–310.

107. Hansen BA, Greiff J, Bergmann F: Fractures of the tibia in children. *Acta Orthop Scand* 1976;47:448–453.

108. Verstreken L, Delronge G, Lamoureux J: Orthopaedic treatment of pediatric multiple trauma patients: A new technique. *Int Surg* 1988;73:177–179.

109. McBryde AM Jr, Blake R: The floating knee—Ipsilateral fractures of the femur and tibia. *J Bone Joint Surg* 1974;56A:1309.

110. Letts M, Vincent N, Gouw G: The "Floating Knee" in children. *J Bone Joint Surg* 1986;68B:442–446.

111. Alonso JE, Horowitz M: Use of the AO/ASIF external fixator in children. *J Pediatr Orthop* 1987;7:594–600.

112. Love SM, Ganey T, Ogden JA: Postnatal epiphyseal development: The distal tibia and fibula. *J Pediatr Orthop* 1990;10:298–305.

113. Kleiger B, Mankin HJ: Fracture of the lateral portion of the distal tibia epiphysis. *J Bone Joint Surg* 1964;46A:25–32.

114. Dias LS, Tachdjian MO: Physeal injuries of the ankle in children; classification. *Clin Orthop* 1978;136:230–233.

115. Lauge-Hansen N: Fractures of the ankle II. Combined experimental-surgical and experimental-roentgenologic investigations. *Arch Surg* 1950;60:957–985.

116. Herzenberg JE: Computed tomography of pediatric distal tibial growth plate fractures: A practical guide. *Techniques Orthop* 1989;4:53–64.

117. Jarvis JC, McIntyre WMJ, England RE: Computerized tomography and the triplane fracture, in Uhthoff HK, Wiley JJ (eds): *Behavior of the Growth Plate*. New York, Raven Press, 1988.

118. Dias LS: Fractures of the tibia and fibula, in Rockwood CA Jr, Wilkins KE, King RE (eds): *Fractures in Children*. Philadelphia, JB Lippincott, 1984, chap 12, pp 983–1042.

119. Mølster A, Søreide O, Solhaug JH, et al: Fractures of the lateral distal tibial epiphysis (Tillaux or Kleiger fracture). *Injury* 1976;8:260–263.

120. Leach RE: Fractures of the tibia and fibula, in Rockwood CA Jr, Green DP (eds): *Fractures in Adults*, ed 2. Philadelphia, JB Lippincott, 1984, chap 17, pp 1593–1663.

121. Kling TF Jr, Bright RW, Hensinger RN: Distal tibial physeal fractures in children that may require open reduction. *J Bone Joint Surg* 1984;66A:647–657.

122. Spiegel PG, Mast JW, Cooperman DR, et al: Triplane fractures of the distal tibial epiphysis. *Clin Orthop* 1984;188:74–89.

123. Letts RM: The hidden adolescent ankle fracture. *J Pediatr Orthop* 1982;2:161–164.

124. Cooperman DR, Spiegel PG, Laros GS: Tibial fractures involving the ankle in children: The so-called triplane epiphyseal fracture. *J Bone Joint Surg* 1978;60A:1040–1046.

125. Marmor L: An unusual fracture of the tibial epiphysis. *Clin Orthop* 1970;73:132–135.

126. Gilmer PW, Herzenberg J, Frank JL, et al: Computerized tomographic analysis of acute calcaneal fracture. *Foot Ankle* 1986;6:184–193.

127. Canale ST, Kelly FB Jr: Fractures of the neck of the talus: Long-term evaluation of seventy-one cases. *J Bone Joint Surg* 1978;60A:143–156.

128. Gross RH: Fractures and dislocations of the foot, in Rockwood CA Jr, Wilkins KE, King RE (eds): *Fractures in Children*. Philadelphia, JB Lippincott, 1984, chap 13, pp 1043–1103.

129. Letts RM, Gibeault D: Fractures of the neck of the talus in children. *Foot Ankle* 1980;1:74–77.

INDEX